HIKE LIST P9-DER-315

MENASHA RIDGE PRESS
Birmingham, Alabama

60 HIKES WITHIN 60 MILES

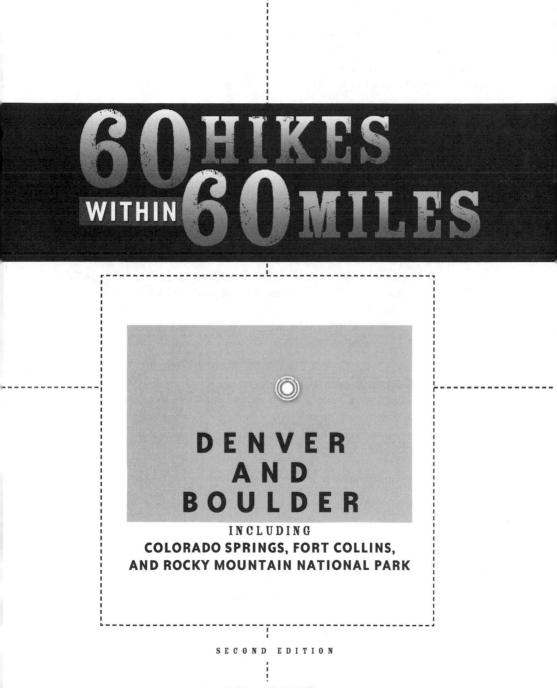

DENVER AND BOULDER

INCLUDING
COLORADO SPRINGS, FORT COLLINS,
AND ROCKY MOUNTAIN NATIONAL PARK

SECOND EDITION

KIM LIPKER

60 Hikes within 60 Miles: Denver and Boulder

Copyright © 2010 by Kim Lipker
All rights reserved
Printed in the United States of America
Published by Menasha Ridge Press
Distributed by Publishers Group West
Second edition, second printing 2011

Library of Congress Cataloging-in-Publication Data

Lipker, Kim, 1969–
   60 hikes within 60 miles, Denver and Boulder : including Colorado
Springs, Fort Collins, and Rocky Mountain National Park / Kim Lipker.
— 2nd ed.
         p. cm.
      Includes bibliographical references and index.
      ISBN-13: 978-0-89732-885-2 (alk. paper)
      ISBN-10: 0-89732-885-X (alk. paper)
         1. Hiking—Colorado—Denver Region—Guidebooks. 2. Denver Region
(Colo.)—Guidebooks. I. Title. II. Title: Sixty hikes within sixty
miles, Denver and Boulder.
                  GV199.42.C62D474 2010
                  796.5109788'83—dc22

                                          2010008280

Cover and text design by Steveco International
Cover photos by Kim Lipker
Author photo copyright Kim Lipker
All other photos by Kim Lipker, Bruce Becker, Michael Bollinger, and Kyle Martin
Maps by Kim Lipker, Ben Pease, and Scott McGrew

Menasha Ridge Press
P.O. Box 43673
Birmingham, AL 35243
www.menasharidge.com

FOR ANNA AND ALEX AND EMMA
LET THE MUSIC OF THE MOUNTAINS DANCE WITHIN YOUR HEART

TABLE OF
CONTENTS

ACKNOWLEDGMENTS

I AM MOST THANKFUL for the fact that I was born in Colorado and that my kids are sixth-generation natives of the state. It's hard to think of living anywhere else. I would also like to thank the following for helping me write the update for this book:

Ron Graham for your unconditional support; Ruth and Roger Lipker for your support and for helping out with the grandkids; Karen Lipker for fact-checking this edition; Anna, Alex, and Emma Lipker for being great kids; Kyle Martin for helping with the new hikes and my REI presentations . . . and to our friend Chad Brent for putting the wheels in motion; Kay Kimball for your consistent enthusiasm for life and my life in particular; to everyone at Menasha Ridge Press, past and present, for everything; Diane Stanko-Martinez and Marty Martinez for true friendship; Geri Kidawski for your expert Master Naturalist guidance and your friendship; Jen Janssen for being the absolute best mom and best friend I will ever know; Johnny Molloy for being a mentor and walking me through your success; Abby Balfany for being the best neighbor, friend, lead support staff, and Team Kim president; Laurel School of Arts & Technology for being a safe, fun place to learn—having my kids at such a terrific neighborhood school feels like an automatic second family; Renee Putman, Kris Baltrum, and Murielle Watzky-Brewer for always being there and for your unwavering support; Nancy Stilson-Herzog for being the trainer extraordinaire; Deb Murr and All Star Cleaning for giving me time at home; and Michael Bollinger, Lindsay Hopper, Lindsay Smith, Lisa Eaton, Kelly Josephs, Fiona Wilson, Suellen May, Jenni, Leslie, Darcy, Old Town Writing Group (Laura, Sarah, Leslie), and Shannon are all people who helped with the first edition of this book and still make their mark.

To the outreach coordinators at the Colorado REI stores: Thank you for continuing to invite me to your stores and for giving me the opportunity to promote hiking and the outdoors.

Thank you to all of my fans and to all of the people who buy my books and attend my clinics and presentations. I am humbled by your support.

Thank you to all the land stewards in Colorado who volunteer to make the hiking here some of the best in the world. There are too many to name. Your tireless efforts make the trails safe and keep them preserved for generations to come.

—Kim Lipker

FOREWORD

Welcome to Menasha Ridge Press's *60 Hikes within 60 Miles,* a series designed to provide hikers with information needed to find and hike the very best trails surrounding cities usually underserved by good guidebooks.

Our strategy was simple: First, find a hiker who knows the area and loves to hike. Second, ask that person to spend a year researching the most popular and very best trails around. And third, have that person describe each trail in terms of difficulty, scenery, condition, elevation change, and all other categories of information that are important to hikers. "Pretend that you've just completed a hike and met up with other hikers at the trailhead," we told each author. "Imagine their questions; be clear in your answers."

An experienced hiker and writer, author Kim Lipker has selected 60 of the best hikes in and around the Denver metropolitan area. From the urban paths of Washington Park to the glaciers of Indian Peaks Wilderness to the prairies of Rocky Mountain Arsenal National Wildlife Refuge, Lipker provides trekkers of all abilities with a great variety of hikes—and all within roughly 60 miles of Denver.

You'll get more out of this book if you take a moment to read the introduction explaining how to read the trail listings. The Topographic Maps section will help you understand how useful topos will be on a hike, and will also tell you where to get them. And though this is a "where-to," not a "how-to" guide, experienced hikers and novices alike will find the introduction of particular value.

As much for the opportunity to free the spirit as well as to free the body, let these hikes elevate you above the urban hurry.

All the best,
The Editors at Menasha Ridge Press

ABOUT THE AUTHOR

KIM LIPKER grew up in Colorado doing most of the hikes featured in this book, never imagining that her frolics through the forest would ever land themselves in print. She grew up in Colorado loving the outdoors from an early age. Kim is the author of four other guidebooks, *The Best in Tent Camping: Colorado, 4th Edition* (with Johnny Molloy for Menasha Ridge Press), *The Unofficial Guide to Bed & Breakfasts and Country Inns in the Rockies* (John Wiley & Sons), *Day and Overnight Hikes: Rocky Mountain National Park* (Menasha Ridge Press), and *Smart and Savvy Hiking: What Every Woman Needs to Know on the Trail* (Menasha Ridge Press). In addition to writing books, Kim writes a regular parenting column and other features for *Rocky Mountain Parent* magazine; for the Web site Away.com, she contributes features, ratings, and reviews covering parks, active sports, and outdoor adventures in the Rocky Mountains and Hawaii.

Considered an expert on the Rocky Mountains by her guidebook peers, Kim has been at the writing thing for a while, having had her first news article published at age 12 and later earning a journalism degree from the University of Missouri–Columbia.

Kim lives in Fort Collins, Colorado, with her family.

For more information on her upcoming projects, visit her blog at **trekalong.com/lipker.**

PREFACE

WRITING A HIKING GUIDEBOOK

Hiking books are tough work. Just kidding! This project enabled me to do two of my favorite things: hike and write. Thanks to a healthy fan base, the 60 Hikes project has been very popular. With all of the input from said fans, we realized that it was time for a rewrite, or a second edition if you will. We have taken the book apart, and this revision entails a complete update of the book. We've done a lot of detailed fact-checking, swapped a few new hikes for ones that might not have held up so well, and selected some new photos. We have a new text design for the guide, along with regional maps, new latitude and longitude material, and updated hiking maps.

It is still quite a challenge to narrow down the hikes in the 60-mile radius into 60 feasible, well-rounded hikes. Boulder County alone has more than 100 hikes to its name. We've hiked every hike in this book, some dozens of times, but we are always mindful of the experienced crowd of hikers in Colorado.

Let me assure you that every hike was chosen for its unique merits. I am the type of person who chooses a wine by how the bottle's label design or wine name pops out at me. Although some of the hiking trails have peculiar names, such as Devil's Backbone Trail in Loveland, I had a more scientific approach to their inclusion. Every trail in Colorado was previewed, narrowed down, and then balanced by skill and region. I consulted hiking clubs and then made final cuts. Every trail is one that I would recommend to my publisher if she visited Denver.

COLORADO FRONT RANGE

Denver is a world-class city with an amazing independent pioneer spirit. Critics have often called Denver a cow town, but rest assured that I've never seen a cow there, save for an old Mr. Steak costume in a St. Patrick's Day parade. Denver's appeal has everything to do with the unique blend of recreational activities available to Colorado's residents and visitors. Where else can you hike a glacier in the morning and go to a Broadway production of *Wicked* downtown in the evening?

For readers unfamiliar with the geography or terminology specific to Denver, here is a quick primer. Denver basically sits in the middle of Colorado at the base of the Rocky Mountains. The state is split in half: to the west are the mountains; to the east are the plains. Fort Collins and Boulder are north of Denver, and Colorado Springs is south. These four cities make a line called the Colorado Front Range.

Weather in this area is usually ten degrees warmer than in the mountains. Summer can be hot and winter cold, but on average, the weather is quite mild and pleasant, and the blue sky blazes with a bright sun almost every day. Don't be surprised if some of the Front Range and foothill towns are windy. Their location on the map leads to some mighty gusts in winter.

Tourist season tends to vary from town to town, but summer is the high season in Estes Park and Rocky Mountain National Park. In the fall, Boulder (home to University of Colorado) and Fort Collins (home to Colorado State University) bustle with college students.

Colorado Springs is the land of "America the Beautiful." The famous song, written by Pikes Peak native Katharine Lee Bates more than a century ago, still speaks volumes about the area, the state, and our country's breathtaking beauty: "spacious skies, amber waves of grain, purple mountains' majesty above the fruited plain." You will understand why this is such an inspiring place when you visit its attractions, from Pikes Peak to Garden of the Gods.

The Eastern Colorado prairie is one of the largest regions in Colorado and one of the least populated. Nothing is hidden in a land that is every bit as dramatic as its mountain-peak cousins. Here are rolling hills, golden fields of wheat, fierce thunderstorms, and threats of tornadoes.

DENVER, COLORADO

This capital city sits at 1 mile above the sea, 5,280 feet to be exact (hence the name mile-high city; 5,280 feet equal one mile). Recent economic growth and population increases have made Denver quite a cosmopolitan city. You'll find new sporting complexes, renovated cultural centers, talented chefs, top-notch shopping, and activities for all ages. This area is home to the state's largest concentration of population and its center of government, commerce, and culture. For the purpose of this book, we have defined greater Denver as the downtown area and the metropolitan area immediately surrounding it.

While Denver is a city looking toward the future, it is also a great place to learn about Colorado's rich history. A host of museums and landmarks pay homage to this wonderful Western heritage: The Denver Art Museum, the Denver

Museum of Natural History, the Colorado History Museum, the Buffalo Bill Museum, the Black American West Museum, and the Molly Brown House are just a few places to visit during your stay.

You can explore both the world and other areas of Colorado in the greater Denver area. Downtown Aquarium features sharks, stingrays, and unique exhibits such as the Indonesian River Journey. More than 3,000 animals call the Denver Zoo home, and Denver Botanic Gardens boasts a wide variety of flowering plants from around the world. Denver averages 300 days of sunshine a year. That's more days of annual sun than in San Diego or Miami Beach. Visitors come to Denver for business and pleasure all year. Dining, theater, special events, and festivals round out a hearty helping of things to do and enjoy in Denver. Perhaps that is why one of four people living in the metro area moved to Denver in the past decade. The city has essentially doubled its population since 1960.

ROCKY MOUNTAIN NATIONAL PARK

The crowning jewel of the 60 hikes is Rocky Mountain National Park. If you travel too far into the park, you miss the 60-mile mark, but you can still find plenty of perimeter hikes to whet your appetite for day and overnight hikes in Rocky Mountain National Park. These hikes include Longs Peak, Gem Lake, Lily Mountain, Storm Pass Trail to Estes Cone, and Twin Sisters.

Visitors to the Front Range will most likely join thousands of others (3 million to be exact) who make their way to Rocky Mountain National Park every year. It is truly an experience not to be missed. It is said that more than 110 mountain peaks tower over the 415 square miles of hiking trails, picnic spots, waterfalls, cold lakes, and bountiful wildlife. I recommend visiting the area in the fall, when the elk are in the valleys for their bugling, or mating, season. Crowds are waning, the colors are changing, and the weather is still quite pleasant.

HISTORY AND A PERSONAL TOUCH

After many years of researching and writing hiking guidebooks, I've learned a lot about the hikes that I really like to do. While I have the physical capability to hike glaciers and the like, I realized that I am actually a bigger fan of moderate loop and balloon trails. While you are perusing the hikes in this book, remember that all hikes are not one-size fits all, and that you need to determine what your comfort level is and what your preferences are and then dig in.

I continue to be impressed by the hikes in Boulder County and Jefferson County, and am so happy at the progress made there, in my old stomping grounds. The trails here are constantly upgraded, and acquiring open space is a priority in both counties.

Lesser-known hikes, such as the urban hikes, were nice to revisit. These urban hikes tend to be easier and less crowded and are a great way to get novice hikers interested in the sport. Washington Park in downtown Denver is a great place to spend a Saturday morning.

The best way to explore the history of Denver and the surrounding area is to visualize those people who have walked the trails before you. Pioneers who just crossed the prairie may have stopped in their wagons to fill water jugs at Barr Lake State Park. A gold miner down on his luck may have found hope near Eldorado Springs Trail.

Native American children may have climbed Arthur's Rock every day. In the 1930s, women who climbed Longs Peak for recreation sometimes had to camp separately from the men and cook their camp dinner. (My grandma was one of them.)

If you are hiking in Estes Park, be sure to stop at the Stanley Hotel. My aunt has waitressed there for many years, and it is rich with stories; they say that Stephen King found the inspiration for *The Shining* while staying there. (If you need a break from hiking, you must try the super haunted hotel tour here.)

There is always the bad with the good, and the biggest bad goes to the little boy who hit my pregnant friend in the stomach while passing us in Meyer Ranch Open Space. It was also annoying to see so many hikers with their dogs off the leash and not picking up their dog's poop. Be warned: Many places ticket hikers if they don't follow the rules, which are there for a reason. A friend of a friend got a heavy fine for having her dog off of the leash on the Meyers Homestead Trail.

In the time that it took me to research and write the first edition of this book, a forest ranger died while hiking in Rocky Mountain National Park, another experienced hiker was lost and then found in the same park, and a man was allegedly mugged at a Jefferson County trailhead. While working on this new edition, two women who were hiking were attacked by a man wielding a knife. They credit their escape to being together and to having a hiking stick, which they used in their defense. This just serves as a reminder to please be careful on the trail and always hike with a buddy. At the very least, let someone know where you are going and when you expect to be back.

Thank you for picking up this book. Be assured that I had you, the reader, in mind during every one of my hikes.

HIKING RECOMMENDATIONS

HIKES 1 TO 3 MILES

HIKES 3 TO 6 MILES

HIKES 3 TO 6 MILES (*continued*)

HIKES 6 TO 9 MILES

HIKES LONGER THAN 9 MILES

TRAILS WHERE SOME PORTION IS GOOD FOR CHILDREN, NOVICES, AND THE OLDER SET

HIKES FOR KIDS

HIKES FOR KIDS (*continued*)

TRAILS FOR HARD-CORE HIKERS

TRAILS WHERE SOME PORTION IS CONCRETE OR ASPHALT

TRAILS GOOD FOR DOGS

MOSTLY FLAT HIKES

HIKES WITH STEEP SECTIONS

ALPINE HIKES

HIKES ALONG WATER

PLENTIFUL-WILDLIFE HIKES

GOOD WINTER HIKES

(Remember to check weather conditions first; winters in Colorado are fickle.)

2. Boulder: Heil Valley Ranch (page 22)
4. Boulder: South Boulder Creek Trail (page 30)
5. Boulder: Walden Ponds (page 34)
6. Chautauqua Park: Royal Arch (page 37)
7. Eldorado Canyon: Eldorado Springs Trail (page 41)
13. Walker Ranch: Meyers Homestead Trail (page 64)
14. Alderfer Three Sisters Open Space Park: Ponderosa Sisters Loop (page 70)
15. Barr Lake State Park: Lake Perimeter Trail (page 73)
16. Bear Creek Lake Park: Bear Creek Trail (page 77)
17. Deer Creek Open Space Park: Meadowlark Plymouth Creek Loop (page 80)
18. Denver: Washington Park (page 83)
19. Elk Meadow Open Space Park: Sleepy S Loop (page 86)
22. Lakewood: Green Mountain and Hayden Trail Loop (page 96)
23. Meyer Ranch Open Space Park: Lodgepole Loop (page 99)
28. Red Rocks: Trading Post Trail (page 114)
29. Rocky Mountain Arsenal National Wildlife Refuge: Lakes Loop (page 118)
30. Westminster: Colorado Hills Trail (page 121)
31. White Ranch Park: Belcher Hill (page 124)
33. Cathy Fromme Prairie: Fossil Creek Trail (page 134)
35. Horsetooth Mountain Open Space: Horsetooth Falls and Horsetooth Rock (page 141)
36. Larimer County: Devil's Backbone Trail (page 145)
38. Lory State Park: Arthur's Rock (page 152)
39. Rabbit Mountain: Eagle Wind Trail (page 156)
40. Rocky Mountain National Park: Gem Lake (page 160)
47. Blodgett Peak Open Space: Water Tank Trail (page 188)
48. Castlewood Canyon State Park: Inner Canyon Loop (page 191)
50. Douglas County Open Space: Glendale Farm Trail (page 197)
51. Douglas County Open Space: Greenland Trail (page 200)
52. Florissant Fossil Beds: Petrified Forest Loop (page 203)
53. Garden of the Gods: Perkins Central Garden Trail (page 207)
54. North Cheyenne Cañon Park: Lower Columbine Trail (page 210)
57. Pine Valley Ranch Park: Pine Valley Ranch Loop (page 219)
58. Reynolds Open Space Park: Raven's Roost Oxen Draw Loop (page 222)
59. Roxborough State Park: South Rim Trail (page 225)
60. Waterton Canyon Recreation Area: Waterton Canyon (page 228)

FOOT-TRAFFIC-ONLY HIKES

(This usually means no bikes, no horses, and no motorized vehicles.)

GEOLOGICAL HIKES

TRAILS THAT ARE PARTLY WHEELCHAIR ACCESSIBLE

TRAILS THAT BAN DOGS

HIKES THAT MY 93-YEAR-OLD GRANDPA WOULD HAVE ENJOYED

HIKES THAT MY 93-YEAR-OLD GRANDPA
WOULD HAVE ENJOYED (*continued*)

60 HIKES
WITHIN 60 MILES

DENVER
AND
BOULDER

INCLUDING
COLORADO SPRINGS, FORT COLLINS,
AND ROCKY MOUNTAIN NATIONAL PARK

INTRODUCTION

Welcome to *60 Hikes within 60 Miles: Denver and Boulder.* If you're new to hiking or even if you're a seasoned trailsmith, take a few minutes to read the following introduction. We explain how this book is organized and how to use it.

HIKE DESCRIPTIONS

Each hike contains seven key items: a brief description of the trail, a key at-a-glance information box, directions to the trail, a trail map, an elevation profile, a more detailed trail description, and a description of nearby activities. Combined, the maps and information provide a clear method to assess each trail from the comfort of your favorite reading chair.

IN BRIEF

A taste of the trail. Think of this section as a snapshot focused on the historical landmarks, beautiful vistas, and other sights that you may encounter on the trail.

KEY AT-A-GLANCE INFORMATION

The information in the key at-a-glance boxes gives you a quick idea of the specifics of each hike. Thirteen basic elements are covered.

LENGTH The length of the trail from start to finish. There may be options to shorten or extend the hikes, but the mileage corresponds to the described hike. Consult the hike description to help decide how to customize the hike for your ability or time constraints.

CONFIGURATION A description of what the trail looks like from overhead. Trails can be loops, out-and-backs (trails on which one enters and leaves along the same path), figure eights, or balloons (trails on which one enters and leaves on the same path with a loop in between).

1

DIFFICULTY The degree of effort an "average" hiker should expect on a given hike. For simplicity, difficulty is described as "easy," "moderate," or "difficult."

SCENERY A rating of the overall environs of the hike and what to expect in terms of plant life, wildlife, streams, and historic buildings.

EXPOSURE A quick check of how much sun you can expect on your shoulders during the hike. Descriptors used include terms such as "shady," "exposed," and "sunny."

TRAFFIC Indicators of how busy the trail might be on an average day, and if you might be able to find solitude out there. Trail traffic, of course, varies from day to day and season to season.

TRAIL SURFACE A description of the trail surface, be it paved, rocky, dirt, or a mixture of elements.

HIKING TIME The length of time it takes to hike the trail. A slow but steady hiker will average 2 to 3 miles an hour, depending on the terrain. Most of the estimates in this book reflect a speed of about 2 miles per hour. Take the miles of the hike and divide by two and this will give a rough estimate of hiking time. For example, an 8-mile hike should take the average hiker four hours.

SEASON The best months to hike the trail determined by access and weather conditions.

ACCESS A notation of fees or permits needed to access the trail (if any) and whether the trail has specific hours.

MAPS Which maps are the best, or easiest, for this hike and where to get them.

FACILITIES What to expect in terms of restrooms, phones, water, and other amenities available at the trailhead or nearby.

SPECIAL COMMENTS These comments cover little extra details that don't fit into any of the above categories. Here you'll find information on trail-hiking options and facts, or tips on how to get the most out of your hike.

DIRECTIONS TO THE TRAIL

The detailed directions will lead you to each trailhead. If you use GPS technology, provided latitude and longitude and UTM coordinates allow you to navigate directly to the trailhead.

TRAIL DESCRIPTIONS

The trail description is the heart of each hike. Here, the author provides a summary of the trail's essence and highlights any special traits the hike offers. Ultimately, the hike description will help you choose which hikes are best for you.

NEARBY ACTIVITIES

Look here for information on nearby hikes.

MAPS

THE OVERVIEW MAP AND KEY

Use the overview map on the inside front cover to find the exact location of each hike's primary trailhead. Each hike's number appears on the overview map, on the hike list facing the overview map, and in the table of contents. As you flip through the book, you'll see that a hike's full profile is easy to locate by watching for the hike number at the top of each page. The book is organized by region as indicated in the table of contents. A map legend that details the symbols found on trail maps appears on the inside back cover.

REGIONAL MAPS

The book is divided into regions, and prefacing each regional section is an overview map of that region. The regional map provides more detail than the overview map does, bringing you closer to the hike.

TRAIL MAPS

Each hike contains a detailed map that shows the trailhead, route, significant features, facilities, and topographic landmarks such as creeks, overlooks, and peaks. The author gathered map data by carrying Garmin eTrex or Garmin 60CS GPS units while hiking. This data was downloaded into the digital mapping program Topo USA and processed by expert cartographers to produce the highly accurate maps found in this book. Each trailhead's GPS coordinates are included with each profile (see below).

ELEVATION PROFILES

Each hike contains a detailed elevation profile that corresponds directly to the trail map. The elevation profile provides a quick look at the trail from the side, enabling you to visualize how it rises and falls. Note the number of feet between each tick mark on the vertical axis (the height scale). To avoid making flat hikes look steep and steep hikes appear flat, height scales are used throughout the book to provide an accurate assessment of each hike's climbing difficulty.

GPS TRAILHEAD COORDINATES

In addition to highly specific trail outlines, this book also includes the GPS coordinates for each trailhead in two formats: latitude/longitude and UTM. Latitude/longitude coordinates tell you where you are by locating a point west (latitude) of the 0° meridian line that passes through Greenwich, England, and north or south of the 0° (longitude) line, also known as the equator, that belts the Earth.

Topographic maps show latitude/longitude as well as UTM grid lines. Known as UTM coordinates, the numbers index a specific point using a grid method. The survey datum used to arrive at the coordinates in this book is WGS84 (versus NAD27 or WGS83). For readers who own a GPS unit, whether handheld or onboard a vehicle, the latitude/longitude or UTM coordinates provided on the first page of each hike may be entered into the GPS unit. Just make sure your GPS unit is set to navigate

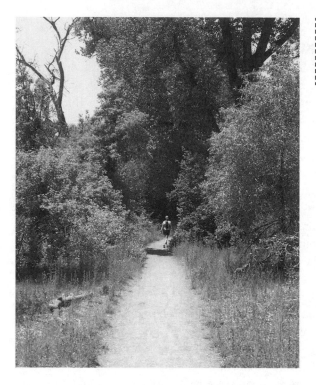

using WGS84 datum. Now you can navigate directly to the trailhead.

Most trailheads, which begin in parking areas, can be reached by car, but some trailheads are a short walk from a parking area. In those cases a handheld unit is necessary to continue the GPS navigation process. That said, readers can easily access all trailheads in this book by using the directions given, the overview map, and the trail map, which shows at least one major road leading into the area. But for those who enjoy using the latest GPS technology to navigate, the necessary data has been provided. A brief explanation of the UTM coordinates from the Eldorado Springs Trail on page 41 follows.

UTM Zone (WGS84) 13S

Easting   0474939

Northing   4419936

The UTM zone number **13** refers to one of the 60 vertical zones of the Universal Transverse Mercator (UTM) projection. Each zone is 6 degrees wide. The UTM zone letter **S** refers to one of the 20 horizontal zones that span from 80° south to 84° north. The easting number **0474939** indicates in meters how far east or west a point is from the central meridian of the zone. Increasing easting coordinates indicate that you are moving east; decreasing easting coordinates indicate that you are moving west. Since lines of longitude converge at the poles, they are not parallel as lines of latitude are. This means that the distance between full easting coordinates is 1,000 meters near the equator but becomes smaller as you travel farther north or south. The difference is small enough to be ignored, but only until you reach the polar regions.

The northing number **4419936** references in meters how far you are from the equator. Above and below the equator, increasing northing coordinates indicate that you are traveling north; decreasing northing coordinates indicate that you are traveling south. To enhance your outdoor experiences with GPS technology, refer to *GPS Outdoors: A Practical Guide for Outdoor Enthusiasts* (Menasha Ridge Press).

The maps in this book have been produced with great care and, used with the hiking directions, will direct you to the trail and help you stay on course. However, you will find superior detail and valuable information in the United States Geological Survey's 7.5-minute series topographic maps. Topo maps are available online in many locations. The easiest single Web resource is located at **msrmaps.com.** You can view and print topos of the entire United States there, and view aerial photographs of the same area. The downside to topos is that most of them are outdated, having been created 20 to 30 years ago. But they still provide excellent topographic detail.

If you're new to hiking, you might be wondering, "What's a topographic map?" In short, a topo indicates not only linear distance but also elevation, using contour lines. Contour lines spread across the map like dozens of intricate spiderwebs. Each line represents a particular elevation, and at the base of each topo, a contour's interval designation is given. If the contour interval is 200 feet, then the distance between each contour line is 200 feet. Follow five contour lines up on the same map, and the elevation has increased by 1,000 feet.

Let's assume that the 7.5-minute series topo reads "contour interval 40 feet," that the short trail we'll be hiking is two inches in length on the map, and that it crosses five contour lines from beginning to end. What do we know? Well, because the linear scale of this series is 2,000 feet to the inch (roughly two and three-quarters inches representing 1 mile), we know our trail is approximately four-fifths of a mile long (2 inches are 4,000 feet). But we also know that we'll be climbing or descending 200 vertical feet (5 contour lines are 40 feet each) over that distance. And the elevation designations written on occasional contour lines will tell us if we're heading up or down.

In addition to outdoor shops and bike shops, you'll find topos at major universities and some public libraries, where you might try photocopying the ones you need to avoid the cost of buying them. But if you want your own and can't find them locally, visit the United States Geological Survey Web site at **topomaps.usgs.gov.** I also recommend **topozone.com** and others mentioned in the appendix as resources for topographic maps and software.

WEATHER

I must stress that the weather in Colorado can change every ten minutes. Be prepared for anything: sun, snow, flash flood, lightning, and hail. Start by knowing the weather forecast and the road conditions, and pack smart. It can be quite a lovely day in Denver, but a trailhead may be inaccessible due to blizzard conditions. You must be prepared, and you should consider carrying a hiking card (CORSAR, discussed below). If you need to be rescued, these hiking cards can save your life and your pocketbook.

ROAD CONDITIONS

Colorado Traffic Management Center of CDOT
cotrip.org; (303) 639-1111

Colorado Avalanche Information Center
geosurvey.state.co.us/avalanche; (303) 499-9650

CLIMATE OVERVIEW:

Semiarid   Short springs
Dry summers   Mild winters, except in the mountains

AVERAGE HIGHS AND LOWS IN DENVER (degrees Fahrenheit)						
	JAN	FEB	MAR	APR	MAY	JUN
HIGH	43°	47°	52°	62°	71°	81°
LOW	16°	20°	26°	35°	44°	52°
	JUL	AUG	SEP	OCT	NOV	DEC
HIGH	88°	86°	77°	66°	53°	45°
LOW	52°	57°	48°	36°	25°	17°

It is hard to generalize the climate and the altitude throughout Colorado, but what you pack and how you deal with altitude can make or break a hiking trip.

The Rockies' rugged and varied geography creates a number of weather zones. Whatever the region, whatever the season, be sure to dress in layers. In the summer, expect warm days and cool evenings. Bring shorts, hiking boots, a sweater, and a weatherproof jacket. In the winter, bring snow gear for the mountains and warm outerwear for elsewhere.

Denver and most of the hikes in this book sit on the eastern slope of the Continental Divide. The prairie region reaches 4,000 feet above sea level. The tundra and the regions closest to the Continental Divide can reach elevations above 14,000 feet. Keep this in mind when planning your trip.

ALTITUDE SICKNESS

Nothing ruins a hiking trip more often than the body's resistance to altitude adjustment. The illness is usually characterized by vomiting, loss of breath, extreme headache, light-headedness, sleeplessness, and overall flulike aches. My advice: Take it easy. When traveling to a higher altitude, give your body a day or two to adjust to where there is less oxygen, hotter sun, and less air pressure. Drink plenty of water and lay off the alcohol and cigarettes. Wear sunglasses and sunscreen. It's that easy. (As always, if serious symptoms persist, locate the nearest emergency room or call 911.)

HIKING CARD (CORSAR)

The Colorado Outdoor Recreation Search and Rescue Card (CORSAR) may be

purchased at most outdoors shops, such as Recreational Equipment, Inc. (REI). You can buy them for a year for $3 or spend $12 and buy a five-year card. The card is not insurance. It does not pay medical transport, which may include helicopter flights or ground ambulance. The card will allow reimbursement to county sheriffs for costs included on a mission. These costs can include mileage, meals, equipment, gasoline, and rental fees (horses, ATV, aircraft) for vehicles used in the search. By purchasing the card, the CORSAR information says, "you have helped ensure that trained and well-equipped search and rescue teams will respond should you become lost or in need of rescue, and they will not have to incur undue expense due to your emergency."

ALLOCATING TIME

On flat or lightly undulating terrain, I averaged 2 miles per hour when hiking. That speed drops in direct proportion to the steepness of a path, and it does not reflect the many pauses and forays off trail in pursuit of yet another view or place to stop for a snack. Give yourself plenty of time. Few people enjoy rushing through a hike, and fewer still take pleasure in hiking after dark. Remember, too, that your pace naturally slackens over the back half of a long trek.

WATER

"How much is enough? One bottle? Two? Three?! But think of all that extra weight!" Well, one simple physiological fact should convince you to err on the side of excess when it comes to deciding how much water to pack: A hiker working hard in 90° heat needs approximately ten quarts of fluid every day. That's two and a half gallons—12 large water bottles or 16 small ones. In other words, pack along one or two bottles even for short hikes.

For most people, the pleasures of hiking make carrying water a relatively minor price to pay to remain healthy. If you're tempted to drink "found" water, do so only if you understand the risks involved. Probably the most common waterborne "bug" that hikers face is giardia, which may not hit until one to four weeks after ingestion. It will have you passing noxious rotten-egg gas, vomiting, shivering with chills, and living in the bathroom. But there are other parasites to worry about, including E. coli and cryptosporidium (and they are harder to kill than giardia). Better yet, hydrate prior to your hike, carry (and drink) six ounces of water for every mile you plan to hike, and hydrate after the hike.

WHAT TO PACK: FIRST-AID KIT AND HIKER'S ESSENTIALS

Be sure that each hiker has the Forest Service ten essentials, which include a map, compass, water, knife, waterproof matches, high-energy food, suitable extra clothing (such as rain gear), mirror, first-aid kit, and whistle. A first-aid kit may contain more items than you might think. The next page lists just the basics.

- Ace bandages or Spenco joint wraps
- Antibiotic ointment (Neosporin or the generic equivalent)
- Aspirin or acetaminophen
- Band-Aids
- Benadryl or the generic equivalent, diphenhydramine (an antihistamine, in case of allergic reactions)
- Butterfly-closure bandages
- Epinephrine in a prefilled syringe (for those known to have severe allergic reactions to such things as bee stings—available by prescription)
- Gauze and compress pads (one roll and a half-dozen 4-by-4-inch pads)
- Hydrogen peroxide or iodine
- Insect repellent
- Matches or a pocket lighter
- Moleskin or Spenco Second Skin
- Snakebite kit
- Sunscreen
- Water purification tablets or water filter (see "Water" on previous page)
- Whistle (more effective at signaling rescuers than your voice)

The following items are optional but worth their weight:

- Aluminum foil
- Bandanna
- Cellular phone (emergencies only)
- Digital camera
- Disinfectant wipes
- Doggy pickup bags
- Extra batteries
- Flashlight
- Foam pad (for lightning strikes)
- Garbage bag
- Gloves (for warmth)
- GPS receiver
- High-energy food and drinks
- Leash
- Lip balm
- Long pants
- Plastic bags with zip closure
- Raincoat and rain pants
- Shorts
- Socks
- Sunglasses
- Toilet paper
- Watch

HIKING WITH CHILDREN

Hiking with kids can be a great way to introduce them to insects, leaves, pinecones, and wind. It's also wonderful exercise and an even better family-bonding experience. It's time away from laundry, cell phones, and dishes—just you, the kids, and nature.

PLANNING AND PACING

It is not advisable to take newborns out in the wild, but short walks in a stroller or a baby carrier are wonderful sensory and bonding opportunities. When my babies cried, I'd walk around our yard and point out leaves, trees, flowers, and birds. It calmed them and was a great way to build up to longer jaunts.

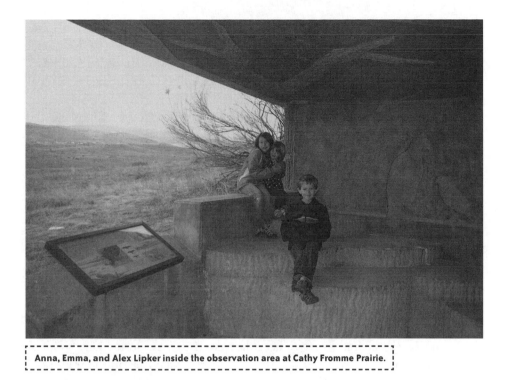

Anna, Emma, and Alex Lipker inside the observation area at Cathy Fromme Prairie.

For children up to age 2, plan to pick them up or strap them in. Baby backpacks, baby carriers, strollers, bike trailers, and more all provide baby and parent with ample opportunity to get on the trail. Paved trails and well-maintained gravel trails all provide access to the younger set.

Children ages 2 to 4 can usually hike up to 2 miles. Be sure to plan plenty of extra time and know that you may end up carrying them. Children ages 5 to 7 can hike 3 to 4 miles over easy terrain. Resting, stopping, and plenty of wandering should be allowed for these age groups. Above age 8, children can easily hike a full day at a slow pace. A full day may include covering 6 miles over variable terrain. Set your entire group or family hiking goals based on the youngest child's ability. Preteens and teenagers may begin to hike more difficult trails if they have had hiking experience.

WHAT TO BRING

Packing for the kids is much like packing for the parents. Be sure that each hiker has the Forest Service ten essentials, which include a map, compass, water, knife, waterproof matches, high-energy food, suitable extra clothing (such as rain gear), mirror, first-aid kit, and whistle. Mom and Dad may want to carry the bulk of the weight and carry obvious things such as the knife and matches. However, as kids can carry more, they will enjoy the responsibility. Make a big deal about buying a small backpack for them to carry their own stuff. This gives the kids ownership of the process, and parents don't end up schlepping it all around.

When hiking with a stroller or other apparatus, it's easy to stash extra essentials such as diapers and baby wipes. Consider packing my list of additional ten kid essentials for the trail: your child's favorite wholesome snack, juice, sunglasses, sunscreen, baby wipes, kid's trail map, kid's magnifying glass, scavenger hunt cards, lunch, and permanent markers.

Be sure that everyone is dressed for the weather. For hot or cold days, the rule is to dress in layers. Start out with more in the winter and less in the summer. All children need to have one proper pair of socks and one proper pair of shoes. Be sure that there is no cotton in the socks, since cotton retains moisture and helps create blisters. Instead, buy child-sized wool socks and nylon liners—there are many different weights and variations for any condition. Good tennis shoes are great, and child-sized hiking boots are even better.

SAFETY CONSIDERATIONS

Children should be taught from the get-go that they must stay within eyesight of an adult. They are to never run ahead on the trail. They are to *never* hike off of the trail. Not only can they get lost or injured, but they can also cause damage to the trail. Teach your kids to treat the outdoors kindly and the outdoors will repay the favor. Teach children to stay where they are if they get lost. Many children relate to *hugging a tree* when lost. Instruct them to find a tree on the trail, hold on, and blow their whistle. Three whistle blows is the standard distress signal and indicates that you are lost or need help. Kids are *never* to go near steep cliffs and other drop-off areas. Rules about rivers and other water sources and climbing on accessible rocks must be addressed. My rule is *no!*

Always teach trail etiquette: Leave no trace, pick up after others who do not, the uphill hiker has the right of way, and don't pick or pull anything. And of course, leaves of three, let them be.

KEEP IT FUN

Before you leave home, have the kids help make a special kid-friendly map that they can keep in their bag. Making maps helps teach direction and creativity. Create a kid-friendly legend that has items such as waterfalls, trails, trees, or rest areas. Draw the route and have the child mark interesting waypoints while they are hiking.

Toy stores are home to many hiking or backyard camping things such as kid's magnifying glasses. A magnifying glass can be used to identify plants, insects, minerals in rocks, and flowers.

Make scavenger-hunt cards to use on any hike. A stack of index cards works fine. Have your child cut hiking-related items from used magazines and paste them on each card. If your child can draw, this works as well. Write the name under the item and bring as many as you want on the trail. You can prolong your scavenger-hunt cards throughout the summer by simply marking each item that you see on the back. It's fun to have a trump card that could be tucked away for special sightings: a bull snake, a lost watch, or an abandoned sock. Bring a permanent marker to take notes on your cards—some may even want to laminate their cards.

Play games like I Spy, try bird-watching, look for animal tracks, or simply count rocks as you hike. The key is to play games that encourage children to observe their surroundings.

Assign a hiking leader (or mountain leader as we call it) and have that child guide the hike. Plan on taking a lot of breaks, and at each break, change the hiking leader. Have your child invite a friend, which helps your child see the world from another youngster's perspective.

If the hike is going well, be sure to head home a little early, especially if you have to turn around and trace your steps. It is always better to end early on a positive note than to end with sore feet, a lot of whining, and discouraged hikers.

HIKING WITH DOGS

I loved hiking with my dog, Bailey. She had a doggy version of ACL surgery during my work on this book, so her mobility was limited. On easy hikes, I'd take her, strap her doggy pack on, and head out. Dogs on trails can lead to some heavy controversy, so use these basic guidelines when taking your hound into the wild.

- **Leashing a dog is the only way to prevent it from chasing wildlife and other trail users. Horses have right-of-way around dogs. A six-foot leash will give your dog enough room to tackle the trail without getting tangled in underbrush or other hikers.**

- **Leashing a dog keeps them from drinking out of streams and other water sources. Harmful bacteria, such as giardia, is a threat to dogs as well as humans. Always pack water for your dog. I use a collapsible doggy bowl and make Bailey carry her own supply of water. A healthy dog should be able to carry up to a third of his weight in a special dog pack.**

- **Leashing dogs keeps them from getting lost. They are also protected from wildlife attacks when on a leash. Nothing is worse than taking a dog to the veterinarian on a weekend with porcupine quills lodged in its sinuses.**

- **Dogs must be in shape before undertaking a hike. Start off small, then work up to longer hikes. Make sure that all of your dog's vaccinations and medications are current, including rabies, bordetella, and heartworm. If you are hiking in an area with Lyme disease, ask your vet about vaccinations.**

- **Keep your dog's paws protected if trails are cold and icy. Bailey has had the hair between her paws become encrusted with ice.**

- **After a hike, carefully check for ticks and burrs. Prepare for accidents and keep antibiotic cream and self-sticking bandage tape in your first-aid kit.**

- **It's essential to pack out dog poop rather than leaving it on the trail or even by the side of the trail. Dog poop is not the same as that of other animals, even that of coyotes or wolves. It's dangerous to the environment, especially** near water sources, and it makes a bad impression on other hikers—not to mention their boots.

- Boulder has a Voice and Sight Control program that says dogs can be off leash, but must stay within your sight and under your control. This means that when you command your dog to come, it does so the first time. You must have a leash for each dog with you. Only two dogs (per person) may be off leash at once. Each dog must display a Voice and Sight dog tag. Everyone who walks the dog on Boulder Open Space Mountain Property must be registered with the Voice and Sight Dog Tag Program. Register with Open Space and Mountain Parks and purchase tags: $15 Boulder resident, includes one tag, and $18.75 nonresident. Additional tags are $5 each.

Special dog note: Pit bulls are not allowed in the city and county of Denver. Owning a pit bull, or bringing one into the city limits, is illegal.

LIGHTNING AND TORNADOES

Get an early start on all hikes that go above tree line. Violent storms are common in June, July, and August. Try to reach high-altitude summits by 1 p.m. and turn back when the weather turns bad. If you are caught in a lightning storm above tree line, stay off ridgetops, spread out if you are in a group, and squat or sit on a foam pad with your feet together. Keep away from rock outcrops and isolated trees. If someone has been struck, be prepared to use CPR to help restore breathing and heartbeat.

In the event of a tornado (they are extremely common in the eastern portion of Colorado), immediately seek shelter. If you are in an open field, lay down in the nearest ditch.

HYPOTHERMIA

Hypothermia occurs when your core body temperature is dangerously low. This condition can occur at any time of the year, and cold temperatures, wind, rain, and snow set the stage for complications. Look for signs of shivering, loss of coordination, and loss of judgment. Prevention in the form of preparation is your best defense against getting cold to the core. Remember the mantra "wet is not warm" to prevent hypothermia. Keep your inside layer as dry as possible.

SNAKES

Spend some time hiking in Denver and you may be surprised by the variety of snakes in the area. Most snake encounters will be with garter snakes, water snakes, and bull snakes (while not venomous, they are rather large and scary-looking). The only venomous snake in the Denver region is the rattlesnake. Rattler sightings are very common. A good rule of thumb is to give them a wide berth and leave them alone. If you are bitten by a rattlesnake, stay calm and get help immediately.

On a side note, my husband was bitten by a rattlesnake in 1999. He was hiking, *alone*, and felt a slap on his leg. Luckily, hikers found him and a search-and-rescue team was deployed. To this day, the old wives' tale holds true: Mosquito bites do not affect him at all. It has long been told that when a person is bitten by a rattlesnake and the venom enters their system, an antibody is released and is always present. Somehow, this antibody acts as a buffer against mosquito venom. When a mosquito bites a past rattlesnake-bite victim, the mosquito venom does not affect them, and thus there is no irritation, bump, or itching.

TICKS

Ticks often wait on brush and tall grass to hitch a ride on a warm-blooded passerby. While they're most visible in the Denver area in early and midsummer, you should be on the lookout for them throughout spring, summer, and fall. Among the local varieties of ticks, deer ticks and dog ticks can transmit diseases. Both of these ticks need several hours of attachment before they can transmit any harbored diseases. Deer ticks, the primary carrier of Lyme disease, are very small, sometimes the size of a poppy seed. You can use several strategies to reduce your chances of ticks getting under your skin. Some people choose to wear light-colored clothing, so ticks can be spotted before they make it to the skin. Insect repellent containing DEET is known as an effective deterrent. Most important, though, be sure to check yourself at the end of the hike. And if it's prime tick season, you may want to perform a quick check every hour or so. For ticks that are already embedded, removal with tweezers is best.

POISON IVY

POISON IVY

Recognizing and avoiding contact with poison ivy is the most effective way to prevent the painful, itchy rashes associated with this plant. Poison ivy occurs as a vine or ground cover with three leaflets to a leaf. Thus the saying: Leaves of three, let them be. Urushiol, the oil in the sap of these plants, is responsible for the rash. Within 12 to 14 hours of exposure, raised lines and/or blisters will appear, accompanied by a terrible itch. Refrain from scratching because bacteria under fingernails can cause infection. Wash and dry the rash thoroughly, then apply a calamine lotion to help dry out the rash. If itching or blistering is severe, seek medical attention. If you do come in contact with one of these plants, remember that oil-contaminated clothing, pets, or hiking gear can easily cause an irritating rash on you or someone else, so wash not only any exposed parts of your body but also clothing, gear, and pets if applicable.

MOSQUITOES

While not common, humans can become infected with the West Nile virus by an infected mosquito. Culex mosquitoes, the primary variety that can transmit West Nile virus to humans, thrive in urban rather than natural areas. They lay their eggs in stagnant water and can breed in any standing water that remains for longer than five days. Most people infected with West Nile virus have no symptoms of illness, but some may become ill, usually 3 to 15 days after being bitten.

In the Denver area, August and September are the high-risk periods for West Nile virus. At this time of year—and anytime you expect mosquitoes to be buzzing around—you may want to wear protective clothing such as long sleeves, long pants, and socks. Loose-fitting, light-colored clothing is best. Spray clothing with insect repellent. Follow the instructions on the repellent carefully and take extra care with children.

CELL PHONES

Do not ever rely on cell phones in the Rockies. Signals and access are very inconsistent. Check with your cellular service provider before leaving home. Many outdoor enthusiasts rely on GPS (Global Positioning Systems) and other forms of communication in the backcountry. Never, never, never make a social call on your cellular phone on a hiking trail.

BLACK BEARS

There are no definite rules about what to do if you meet a bear. In most cases, the bear will detect you first and leave. If you do encounter a bear, here are some suggestions from the National Park Service:

- **Stay calm.**
- **Move away, talking loudly to let the bear discover your presence.**
- **Back away while facing the bear.**
- **Avoid eye contact.**
- **Give the bear plenty of room to escape; bears will rarely attack unless they are threatened or provoked.**
- **Don't run or make sudden movements; running will provoke the bear, and you cannot outrun a bear.**
- **Do not attempt to climb trees to escape bears, especially black bears. The bear will pull you down by the foot.**
- **Fight back if you are attacked. Black bears have been driven away when people have fought back with rocks, sticks, binoculars, and even their bare hands.**
- **Be grateful that it is not a grizzly bear.**

MOUNTAIN LIONS

Lion attacks on people are rare, with fewer than 12 fatalities in 100 years. Based on observations by people who have come in contact with mountain lions, some patterns are beginning to emerge. Here are more suggestions from the National Park Service:

- Stay calm.
- Talk firmly to the lion.
- Move slowly.
- Back up or stop. Never run because lions will chase and attack.
- Raise your arms. If you are wearing a sweater or coat, open it and hold it wide.
- Pick up children and make them appear larger.
- If the lion becomes aggressive, throw rocks and large objects at it. This is the time to convince the lion that you are not prey and that you are a danger to it. Never crouch down or turn your back to retrieve said items.
- Fight back and try to remain standing if you are attacked.

TRAIL ETIQUETTE

Whether you're on a city, county, state, or national park trail, always remember that great care and resources (from nature as well as from your tax dollars) have gone into creating these trails. Treat the trail, wildlife, and fellow hikers with respect.

- Hike on open trails only. Respect trail and road closures (ask if not sure), avoid possible trespassing on private land, and obtain all permits and authorization as required. Also, leave gates as you found them or as marked.
- Leave only footprints. Be sensitive to the ground beneath you. This also means staying on the existing trail and not blazing any new trails. Be sure to pack out what you pack in. No one likes to see the trash someone else has left behind.
- Never spook animals. An unannounced approach, a sudden movement, or a loud noise startles most animals. A surprised snake or skunk can be dangerous to you, to others, and to themselves. Give animals extra room and time to adjust to your presence.
- Plan ahead. Know your equipment, your ability, and the area where you are hiking—and prepare accordingly. Be self-sufficient at all times; carry necessary supplies for changes in weather or other conditions. A well-executed trip is a satisfaction to you and to others.
- Be courteous to other hikers, bikers, or equestrians you meet on the trails.

Boulder (Including Foothills and Mountains)

N

0   3   6
miles

287

Panama Reservoir

Lafayette

287

36

Bloomfield

42

Standley Lake

119

52

95th St.

Niwot

Gunbarrel

Boulder Reservoir

75th St.

5

Left Hand Valley Reservoir

Valmont

119

Valmont Rd.

Leggett Reservoir

Baseline Rd.

Boulder Rd.

7

Baseline Reservoir

128

Superior

72

Marshall

Marshall Lake

4

Boulder

119

36

170

93

36

93

7

6
8

36

S. St. Vrain Creek

Geer Canyon Rd.

2

3

1

Flagstaff Rd.

13

Gross Reservoir

7

Jamestown

Gold Hill

Sugarloaf

119

Middle Boulder Creek

72

Pinecliffe

Thorodin Mtn.

Burnt Mtn.

72

Beaver Reservoir

Ward

Brainard Lake Rd.

S. St. Vrain Creek

Barker Reservoir

Nederland

CR 130

Rollinsville

119

ROOSEVELT NATIONAL FOREST

72

CR 116

Silver Lake

Island Lake

10

CR 16

St. Vrain Glacier

11

Goose Lake

9

ARAPHO NATIONAL FOREST

Peak Glacier

Arapaho Glacier

12

Continental Divide Trl.

BOULDER
(INCLUDING FOOTHILLS AND MOUNTAINS)

01 BETASSO PRESERVE: CANYON LOOP TRAIL

KEY AT-A-GLANCE INFORMATION

LENGTH: 3.2 miles

CONFIGURATION: Loop

DIFFICULTY: Easy

SCENERY: Meadow, forest, views of the Boulder Valley

EXPOSURE: Sunny in meadow, shaded in south-facing portions

TRAFFIC: Moderate during weekdays, crowded on weekends

TRAIL SURFACE: Hard-packed dirt, loose rocks

HIKING TIME: 2 hours

SEASON: All year (south-facing portions may be icy during winter)

ACCESS: Free; open sunrise to sunset

MAPS: USGS Boulder

FACILITIES: Restroom, picnic areas

SPECIAL COMMENTS: There has been significant conflict between mountain bikers and hikers on this trail, so great lengths have been taken to keep this a multiuse trail. Biking is prohibited on Wednesdays and Saturdays. Bikers are required to travel in a single direction on the trail, which changes monthly. Signs posted will indicate the direction, and hikers are advised to hike in the opposite direction of bike traffic. Dogs must be leashed. Restrooms are unappealing.

IN BRIEF

Canyon Loop Trail is located in Boulder County's historic Betasso Preserve, which was an 1870s mining and sawmill town. This well-maintained hike is easy to find and close to Boulder. Half the trail traverses meadows with Douglas fir trees on north-facing slopes. The rest of the trail is shaded by ponderosa pines and lined with moss-covered boulders.

DESCRIPTION

At the Canyon Loop trailhead sign, veer left and head north into a stand of tall ponderosa pines. Pass a group picnic area at the top of the hill where views to the west greet hikers, and head down through a gate, passing an information sign. Climb a small hill, then descend and travel west into the trees. At the trail marker, head north. You'll cross a gully and then climb a slope.

Betasso Preserve is a geology-enthusiast's wonderland, as it lies in the northeast corner of the Colorado mineral belt. Molten material was forced up to the earth's crust 1.7 billion years ago, and instead of bursting through like lava, it settled just beneath the surface and cooled, forming an igneous rock known as the Boulder Creek granodiorite. The slow

GPS Trailhead Coordinates

UTM Zone (WGS84)   13T

Easting   0470690

Northing   4429330

Latitude   N 40.013662°

Longitude   W 105.343439°

Directions

From Denver, take I-25 north to US 36 toward Boulder. Go west on CO 119, also known as Canyon Boulevard. Travel west for 6.2 miles to Sugarloaf Road (about 2 miles after The Alps Inn). Turn right and be wary of a sharp, blind curve. Follow Sugarloaf Road 1 mile, then turn right on Betasso Road, traveling east. Go 0.5 miles to an open gate on the left. Turn here and follow the road to the Canyon Loop Trail parking area.

N

0   0.1   0.2
mile

Fourmile Canyon Rd.

Fourmile Canyon Creek

meadow

Canyon Loop Trl.

**BETASSO
PRESERVE**

Canyon Loop Trl.

Betasso Rd.

Sugarloaf Rd.

**To
Boulder**

Filtration Plant

8,500

8,000

7,500

7,000

FEET

6,500

6,000

5,500

5,000

4,500

0.5   1   1.5   2   2.5   3   3.2

MILES

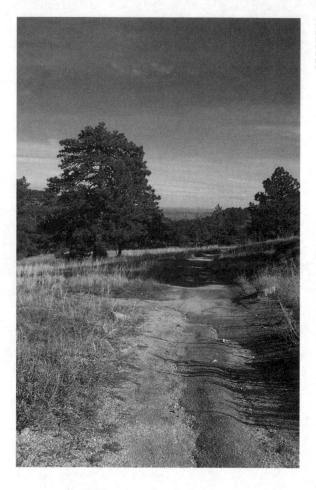

cooling and hardening of this rock formed visible mineral crystals. Boulder Canyon and Fourmile Canyon surround Betasso Preserve, and the forces of erosion are still visible in the spring when the creeks flow through the preserve.

At the top of the hill, head east. A small park bench allows you to sit and catch your breath while enjoying the views of the Boulder Valley and the northern Colorado plains. The meadow blends with the forest, and both host gorgeous wildflowers in the spring and summer.

Pine trees line most of the trail, along with shrubs and grasses. Skunkbrush is the most common shrub. To understand its name, crush one of its delicate twigs and sniff. Not all of the shrubbery in Betasso Preserve is native; cheatgrass, for example, was introduced to the preserve as a result of cattle grazing and now rapidly out-competes native grasses.

After the bench, climb onto a little knoll and then begin to head downhill. The trail circles a knob, where more wonderful views await you, and then winds west along a south-facing slope. Here, you are treated to patches of mysteriously cool air, moss-covered rocks, and thick grasses. Hike through a ravine, then head back east into the woods. Round several switchbacks through several gullies. Even in late summer, these gullies may still hold small, full springs to cross.

Although cattle no longer graze here, many mammals live in Betasso Preserve. You may see mule deer, coyotes, rabbits, and a variety of birds. The Albert's squirrel is common near the picnic area. These squirrels feed on pinecones, and unlike other squirrels, they do not gather and store food for the winter. Instead, they survive the Colorado winter by feeding on the inner bark of pine twigs, and thus are only found where ponderosa pine trees grow.

The staccato drilling of a woodpecker, common at Betasso Preserve, occasionally jars the subtle sounds of the stream, the forest animals, and the breeze rustling through the pines. Continue as the trail bends to the south and then crests a ridge. The trail ascends gently toward the west. At an unmarked trail crossing, go south where the trail reenters the wooded parkland. Reach another natural trail crossing and continue west. Pass a picnic area and turn right on the road. Pass another, larger picnic area near the trailhead and return to the parking lot.

NEARBY ATTRACTIONS

Bummer's Rock Trail, a second trail in Betasso Preserve, and Sugarloaf Mountain Summit Trail. For further information on this area, visit the Web site for the City of Boulder Open Space and Mountain Parks: **bouldercounty.org/openspace.**

02 BOULDER: HEIL VALLEY RANCH

 KEY AT-A-GLANCE INFORMATION

LENGTH: 7.6 miles

CONFIGURATION: Balloon

DIFFICULTY: Moderate

SCENERY: Green valley, ponderosa pines, ranchland, yucca plants, seasonal wildflowers; beautiful views of Longs Peak

EXPOSURE: Little shade

TRAFFIC: Heavy

TRAIL SURFACE: Dirt

HIKING TIME: 4 hours

SEASON: All year

ACCESS: Free; open sunrise to sunset

MAPS: USGS Lyons

FACILITIES: Picnic tables, restrooms, group shelter

SPECIAL COMMENTS: The group shelter accommodates up to 25 people on a first-come, first-serve basis. No groups are permitted on the weekend because of limited parking. This area is popular with mountain bikers, hikers, and equestrians. The 1-mile Lichen Loop, which is not part of this hike, is open to pedestrians only. No dogs are allowed on any of the Heil Valley Ranch trails.

IN BRIEF

Heil Valley Ranch has three trails and is part of Boulder's North Foothills Open Space. The longest trail—and the trail featured here—is the Wapiti Trail combined with the Ponderosa Loop. You'll travel through stands of ponderosa pines and open meadows full of prairie grasses and seasonal wildflowers. Heil Valley Ranch is an important winter range for elk that migrate from Indian Peaks Wilderness—the only herd of elk along the Front Range that migrate from the Continental Divide to the Great Plains. At the turn of the 20th century, elk were eliminated from Boulder County, but they were reintroduced by 1917.

DESCRIPTION

Head straight to the end of the parking area and begin the hike at Wapiti Trail. The trail is singletrack dirt for only 100 feet and then turns into a wide service road. The trail begins in a big, green valley with a lot of tall ponderosa trees. Start a gentle ascent up the valley. The service road crosses through a creek and continues straight. Pass mountain lion warning signs.

Go through an emergency-services gate; pass a spur of the Lichen Loop and take a left after the spur. Continue along the old ranch

GPS Trailhead Coordinates

UTM Zone (WGS84) 13T

Easting   0474450

Northing   4443920

Latitude   N 40.145233°

Longitude W 105.299958°

Directions

From Denver, take I-25 north to US 36 through Boulder. Head toward Lyons and turn left on Lefthand Canyon Road. Travel 0.5 miles and turn right on Greer Canyon Road. Travel 1.3 miles to the Heil Valley Ranch trailhead.

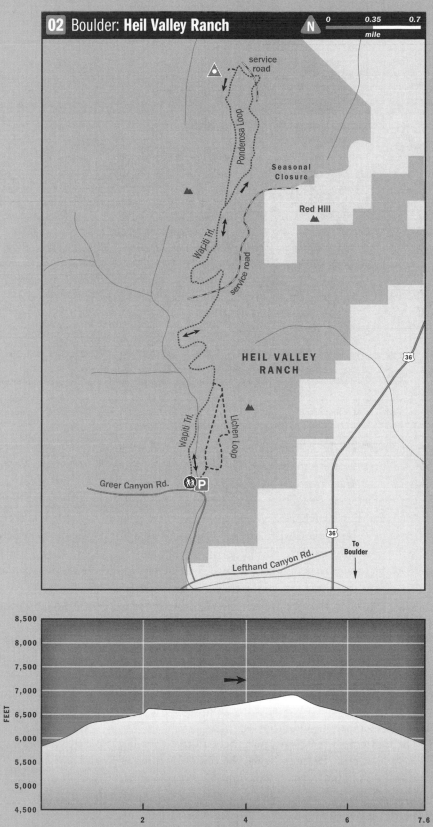

N

0   0.35   0.7

mile

service
road

Ponderosa Loop

Seasonal
Closure

Red Hill

Wapiti Trl.

service road

HEIL VALLEY
RANCH

Wapiti Trl.

Lichen Loop

Greer Canyon Rd.

P

36

To
Boulder

Lefthand Canyon Rd.

36

FEET

8,500

8,000

7,500

7,000

6,500

6,000

5,500

5,000

4,500

2   4   6   7.6

MILES

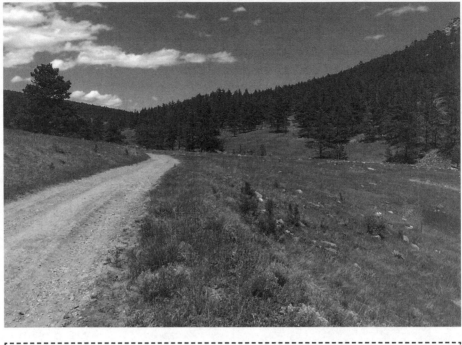

A wide service road is just one of the trail landscapes you will find on the hike at Heil Valley Ranch.

fence that parallels the Wapiti Trail and passes an open meadow and prairie-dog mounds. Notice foothills to the east. The trail is exposed here, but you soon travel into trees. The trail switches to singletrack dirt and crosses a steel-and-wood bridge. Complete one switchback and continue as the trail gets a little rocky.

After another switchback, you eventually enter a lightly forested hillside. Ponderosa trees release a Christmastime pine smell on a hot day as the heat penetrates the needles. Pass through thin grass, yucca plants, and seasonal wildflowers. Cross the service road and keep going. Switchback around the remnants of an old, stone homestead and follow the trail as it goes left.

After 2.5 miles, the Wapiti Trail intersects with the Ponderosa Loop. This is the intersection where the loop part of the balloon hike starts. Continue right, starting a counterclockwise circle, as the trail goes downhill slightly and crosses an open meadow. From here, look right to the expansive views of the Eastern Plains. The trail again travels through a sparse ponderosa forest.

Cross the service road and continue straight. In the distance are old mining relics. Heil Valley Ranch was an early homesteading and mining site. Today it's maintained by ranchers and farmers.

The trail crosses a hillside, meanders a little, then levels out as you begin to approach the top of the loop. Reach the outlook on the right and stop to take in the views west to Longs Peak and Mount Meeker, north to St. Vrain Canyon, and east to the Eastern Plains. Two benches at the overlook provide a nice respite, or find a nice spot to spread a picnic blanket and have lunch.

View of the valley from a higher point of the trail at Heil Valley Ranch.

Past the overlook, the trail becomes scattered with loose rocks as it climbs a gentle grade and remarkably turns to soft beachlike sand. Continue up the hill and the trail will level off, dropping into a flat, open meadow. Pass through a section of young trees in a small meadow. Evidence that workers have made great efforts to maintain the trail is clear here, where they have laid flat stones in the places prone to mud. Start descending as the trail heads back to the intersection of Ponderosa Loop and Wapiti Trail. Get back on the Wapiti Trail and retrace your steps to the trailhead.

03   BOULDER: MOUNT SANITAS

KEY AT-A-GLANCE INFORMATION

LENGTH: 3.36 miles

CONFIGURATION: Loop

DIFFICULTY: Moderate to difficult

SCENERY: Prairie grasses, fir trees, ponderosa trees, wildlife

EXPOSURE: Partly shaded

TRAFFIC: Moderate

TRAIL SURFACE: Hard-packed dirt, loose rocks, some sandy spots

HIKING TIME: 2 hours

SEASON: All year

ACCESS: Free

MAPS: USGS Boulder

FACILITIES: Restroom, pavilion, fire pit, picnic tables

SPECIAL COMMENTS: Dogs must be leashed. Part of the Boulder Voice and Sight Control program. Dogs may be off leash if the green Voice and Sight Control tag is displayed. No bicycles are allowed in this area. Horses are allowed on all trails.

IN BRIEF

Mount Sanitas is a bolder Boulder hike, and access to its challenge is right in town. This hike is an obstacle course of boulders, log and rock steps, steep slabs, and rugged terrain. This is a hike not to be taken lightly, and it is less of a trail and more of a 45-degree free-climb up the side of the mountain. For a good portion of the ascent, the Sanitas Loop has hikers scrambling over boulders and up the side of the sharp sandstone ridges. Mount Sanitas is popular with trail runners, dog lovers, and locals.

DESCRIPTION

Keep watch for the Centennial trailhead, as the Mount Sanitas trailhead is obscured from the road. Parking is provided at the Centennial trailhead or along Mapleton Avenue. A small path leads from the parking lot, across the road, and down some steps to the pavilion with a fire pit and picnic tables. Passing under the pavilion, the trail begins. Go left up the trail to the northwest, and take the wooden stairs to start the ascent. A bridge spans a small stream, and then the trail becomes extremely rocky.

The trail begins on the western side of Mount Sanitas, where the Indian Peaks are in view. Several large rocky outcrops on the left side of the trail offer views to the north

GPS Trailhead Coordinates

UTM Zone (WGS84)   13T

Easting   0474811

Northing   4430017

Latitude   N 40.019984°

Longitude   W 105.295178°

Directions

From Denver, take I-25 north to US 36 to the Baseline Road exit. Take a left turn, going west. Turn right onto Broadway and stay on Broadway for one mile. Turn left onto Mapleton Avenue. Go 0.4 miles past Mapleton Memorial Hospital to the Centennial trailhead parking lot on the left.

03 Boulder: **Mount Sanitas**

N

0   0.1   0.2

mile

S. Cedar Brook Rd.

4th St.

Mt. Sanitas

East Ridge Trl.

Mt. Sanitas Trl.

Sanitas Valley Trl.

Dakota Ridge Trl.

3rd St.

4th St.

5th St.

MORNING SIDE PARK

4th St.

Sunshine Canyon Dr.

stairs

Mt. Sanitas Dr.

BOULDER MOUNTAIN PARK

Alto Ave.

Mapleton Ave.

P

To Boulder and 36

Green Rock Dr.

Sunshine Lake

FEET				
8,500				
8,000				
7,500				
7,000				
6,500				
6,000				
5,500				
5,000				
4,500				

1   2   3   3.36

MILES

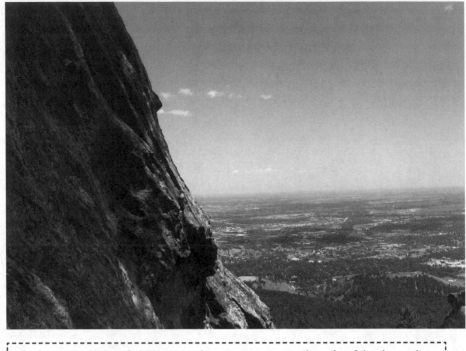

So close to town, yet so far away. Views from Mount Sanitas Trail are plentiful and rewarding.

and south between Mount Sanitas and Indian Peaks. As you ascend farther up the difficult terrain, the trail will flatten slightly as it ascends to the ridge of Mount Sanitas. The first views of Boulder can be seen from a small path that leads to the eastern side of the ridge.

Mount Sanitas was once home to the Sanitas Quarries, named after the Colorado sanitarium started by the Seventh Day Adventists in 1895. The sanitarium eventually became Boulder Memorial Hospital Mapleton Center for Rehabilitation. During the 1920s, the University of Colorado owned and operated the quarries. Many of the older buildings on campus were built from the sandstone pulled from the Sanitas Quarries. The city of Boulder purchased the quarry and surrounding land in 1969, creating a nature and wildlife preserve.

The trail then begins to ascend, crossing back and forth over the ridge of the mountain obscuring Boulder, and then bringing it back into view. The Sanitas Valley Trail can also be seen stretching north and south below. Now the trail stays on top of the ridge, allowing you to see the rest of the mountain. Take advantage of the occasional flat spots, as there will not be a lot of good places to rest farther up the trail.

At this point, the conventional trail is left behind. Toward the summit, the trail is essentially a worn path in the side of the mountain. Hikers are required to scramble over boulders and up sheer rock to progress any farther. Careful footing and handholds become essential because one wrong slip can really hurt. After this final struggle up the last part of the ridge, you finally reach the summit. The summit is rocky and uneven but provides a few areas to take a quick break. Once properly rested and hydrated, you'll begin your descent. A small sign will direct you downward and to the southeast onto East Ridge Trail.

Another small path continues north through a glen of pine trees. The devastation caused by pine beetles is evident as the trail is littered with dead pine needles. This little path takes you through a more densely wooded area and is not nearly as difficult as the Mount Sanitas Loop; however, the path only goes for a little way before a barbed-wire fence stops you from proceeding. At this point, turning back is the only option. It's a nice little trail if you want to take it easy before continuing down the East Ridge Trail.

While not as difficult as the Mount Sanitas Trail, East Ridge Trail offers a lot of the same terrain schemes. It is important to take some time and plan your descent. At several points during this first part of the descent, many large boulders and rocky outcrops hide the trail from view. Take care to notice the small green signs posted on some logs that direct which way to go. Do not stray from these signs. The rocky nature of the terrain means locating any kind of path is extremely difficult. Take your time! Make sure that you know where you're going before you make any hasty decisions. After carefully descending from the boulder-strewn upper altitudes, the trail again becomes a series of rocky steps. While easier to manage than the previous terrain, caution should still be used. The trail then begins to switchback down the east side of the mountain toward the Sanitas Valley.

The switchbacks eventually end as East Ridge Trail meets up with the Sanitas Valley Trail. The Sanitas Valley Trail is a gentle little descent down a well-worn sandy path. Trail runners can be found running up and down this portion of the trail. Sanitas Valley Trail curves around from the north and leads directly south for 1.5 miles to the trailhead. You have two opportunities to hop on Dakota Ridge Trail, which runs parallel with Sanitas Valley Trail for a good portion of the descent. Near the trailhead, a small alcove is to the left, with a shaded area that lies next to the small stream you saw earlier. If you need a place to rest and enjoy a little peace before heading back to the parking lot, this is the perfect place.

NEARBY ATTRACTIONS

City of Boulder Open Space and Mountain Parks: **bouldercounty.org/openspace.**

04   BOULDER:
SOUTH BOULDER CREEK TRAIL

 KEY AT-A-GLANCE INFORMATION

LENGTH: 6.68 miles
CONFIGURATION: Out-and-back
DIFFICULTY: Easy
SCENERY: Open meadow, urban, large creek, mountain views, cottonwoods, prairie grasses
EXPOSURE: Shady along creek
TRAFFIC: Heavy
TRAIL SURFACE: Dirt, some paved portions
HIKING TIME: 3 hours
SEASON: All year
ACCESS: Free; open sunrise to sunset
MAPS: USGS Louisville, Niwot
FACILITIES: Picnic table, grill
SPECIAL COMMENTS: This area is popular with people using wheelchairs, especially sport-equipped chairs. No restroom facilities. Bikes are allowed on the initial part of the trail that is paved (between Baseline Road and East Boulder Community Center). Dogs must be leashed but are not allowed past South Boulder Road to Marshall Road. This makes for a short hike, so you may want to leave the pets at home. As with most Boulder trails, this trail is heavy with bike and pedestrian traffic and a few equestrians, as well.

IN BRIEF

This trail winds southward along a riparian corridor and is highlighted by self-guided interpretive displays. The area offers seasonal viewings of the bobolink, for which the first portion of the trail was named, and other ground nesting birds. Although an urban hike, this trail is a peaceful outing with plenty of wildlife, history, and beauty.

DESCRIPTION

Leave the trailhead and travel south from Baseline Road. The first mile of the trail is soft-surfaced and runs parallel to a paved portion. No bikes are allowed on the soft surface, but hikers may wander back and forth between the two. The soft-surfaced path allows pedestrians to get a little closer to the banks of South Boulder Creek. The trail is well maintained and lined on the west with cottonwood trees and on the east with prairie grasses.

Pass large, old cottonwoods and lush undergrowth that hugs the creek. Travel along a split-rail fence and cross the paved path that has been running parallel to the soft-surfaced trail up until this point. Pass the East Boulder Community Center trail connection to the right as the trail becomes a narrow singletrack, but still very soft, smooth, and flat. The paved

GPS Trailhead Coordinates

UTM Zone (WGS84) 13S
Easting   0481700
Northing 4427520
Latitude N 39.997664°
Longitude W 105.214380°

Directions

From Denver, take I-25 north to US 36, to Foothills Parkway in Boulder. Turn right on Foothills Parkway off of US 36. Travel approximately 1 mile and turn right on Baseline Road. Take Baseline Road east until just before Cherryvale Road. The Bobolink trailhead is just west of the intersection of Baseline and Cherryvale roads.

N

0   0.25   0.5
mile

157

Baseline Rd.

Foothills Pkwy.

Baseline Reservoir

To Boulder

36

Baseline Dam

South Boulder Rd.

S. Cherryvale Rd.

South Boulder Creek Trl.

South Boulder Creek

93

36

To Denver

8,500

8,000

7,500

7,000

6,500

6,000

5,500

5,000

4,500

FEET

0.5   1   1.5   2   2.5   3   3.34

MILES

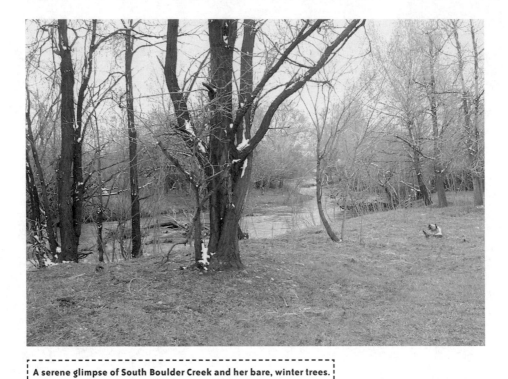

A serene glimpse of South Boulder Creek and her bare, winter trees.

path splits and crosses a bridge that runs over the creek. Hikers continue straight on the soft-surfaced path.

The trail splits away from the creek just before reaching South Boulder Road. Continue and cross a small concrete bridge, then turn left. You will now be going parallel with South Boulder Road. After just a few minutes' walk, you come to another concrete bridge, where you go right. The trail then passes through a tunnel under South Boulder Road.

On the other side of South Boulder Road, come to a gravel road and take a right. Take a left where the creek meets up with the trail again and go through a gate. Be sure to close all gates after you cross through them because livestock roam the fields. Dogs are not allowed south of South Boulder Road because they tend to spook the grazing cows. Cattle are scattered throughout the perimeter of the trail, between South Boulder Road and CO 93, as are their cow patties. A posted sign also warns that the cattle may be aggressive. Ranching is still a part of this area.

Go through another gate, close it, and travel under US 36 via a covered, concrete tunnel. Pass through another gate and be sure to close it. The trail then opens up to a wide, open prairie with views of the Boulder mountains. The noise of US 36 and other roadways is prevalent but not too distracting.

Continue straight all the way to the far end of the field. At the split-rail fence, take a right and go over the boardwalk and through another gate. The prairie is

Cows graze near the trail.

wet and more meadowlike, and is home to deer, nesting birds, and fox. Hikers
continuously travel along the creek, and the creek's shelter makes this urban trail
feel secluded. The trail ends at CO 93, after passing through two more gates and
crossing two more bridges. From here, retrace your steps back to the trailhead.

NEARBY ATTRACTIONS

City of Boulder Open Space and Mountain Parks: **bouldercounty.org/openspace.**

05 BOULDER: WALDEN PONDS

KEY AT-A-GLANCE INFORMATION

LENGTH: 2.5 miles
CONFIGURATION: Loop
DIFFICULTY: Easy
SCENERY: Prairie, ponds, wetland habitat
EXPOSURE: Partly shaded
TRAFFIC: Moderate
TRAIL SURFACE: Dirt, boardwalks
HIKING TIME: 45 minutes
SEASON: All year
ACCESS: Free; open sunrise to sunset
MAPS: USGS Niwot; Walden Ponds map available at trailhead
FACILITIES: Restrooms, picnic tables, shelters, ranger office
SPECIAL COMMENTS: Pick up a field checklist of birds at the trailhead. Fishing is allowed from the shore of the ponds with artificial bait, but wading and boats are prohibited. Leashed dogs are allowed, as are horses and bikes. Special, posted wildlife habitat areas are closed to the public. Many areas of this hike, including a special fishing pier, are wheelchair accessible. Don't be discouraged by the county road maintenance facility with large piles of gravel and a wastewater treatment plant. Beyond this point, the shorelines of the ponds and the views of Indian Peaks are beautiful.

IN BRIEF

The ponds (reclaimed gravel pits) now support a variety of wildlife, including waterfowl, songbirds, and mammals such as beavers, deer, muskrats, and red foxes. The hike around the ponds offers incredible views of the Indian Peaks. Interpretive nature signs along Cottonwood Marsh explain the history and geology of the area. This is a perfect family hike and a nice alternative for those needing accessible trails.

DESCRIPTION

From the parking lot, go left on the trail. On the right you'll see boardwalks that cut through the marshes, which are thick with cattails and prairie grasses. This is the Cottonwood Marsh interpretive trail. If you like, you can take it now or at the end of the hike. The Walden Ponds are a haven for songbirds that can be heard throughout the trail.

After the boardwalk, continue on a gravel trail that parallels a service road. Leave the maintenance facility and gravel piles behind, and enter a land of lush trees, healthy marshes, and boardwalks. Pass Duck Pond on the left and walk toward the ranger field station (open 8 a.m. to 4 p.m., Monday through Friday). The trail turns into a service road and goes past Island Lake and to the right of Bass Pond. Continue straight ahead on the well-marked

GPS Trailhead Coordinates

UTM Zone (WGS84) 13T
Easting   0484355
Northing   4432441
Latitude   N 40.042055°
Longitude W 105.183396°

Directions

From Denver, take I-25 north to US 36 to CO 7 (Arapahoe Avenue) in Boulder. Turn right on CO 7 and travel east for 5 miles to 75th Street. Turn left on 75th Street and travel 2 miles to the entrance of Walden Ponds Open Space. Turn left and park at the Cottonwood Marsh picnic area and trailhead (the second trailhead in the park).

N
0   0.25   0.5
mile

Jay Rd.

Boulder Creek

Heatherwood Trl.

Bass Pond

Pelican Marsh

Island Lake

Cottonwood Marsh

Walden Ponds Entrance Rd.

Interpretive Trl.

P

75th St.

service road

Duck Pond

Sawmill Ponds

To Boulder

Valmont Rd.

FEET

8,500
8,000
7,500
7,000
6,500
6,000
5,500
5,000
4,500

0.5   1   1.5   2   2.5

MILES

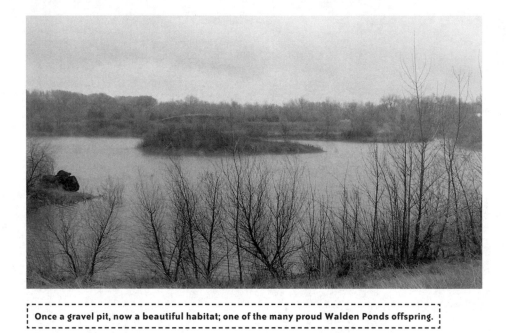

Once a gravel pit, now a beautiful habitat; one of the many proud Walden Ponds offspring.

trail, then bear left around the north side of Bass Pond. On the right is the Heatherwood Trail, which is a paved path offering residential neighborhood access.

Continue counterclockwise around Pelican Marsh. Go left through a fence line to a sign and the first of the Sawmill Ponds. Take a right at the sign and begin a large loop counterclockwise around six of the Sawmill Ponds. The flat trail, sheltered by cottonwood trees, is doubletrack with loose sand and gravel. At the 1-mile mark, the trail bears to the left and into a stand of cottonwood trees. Keep circling around the Sawmill Ponds and savor the views of the Indian Peaks to the west. Look for a large, bleached cottonwood to the right—a favorite hangout for local birds of prey.

At 1.5 miles, the trail curves back toward the east and a bird-watching/viewing blind. At the viewing blind, take a left (going north) and follow the trail along the fence. Duck Pond is on the right, so flip around to the right at the top of Duck Pond and head back east to the parking lot.

Feel free to explore the 51 acres around Walden and Sawmill ponds at any point in the trail. Open pits and puddles of groundwater were all that remained in 1974 after the property had been stripped 15 feet down to bedrock. This will give hikers pause at the beauty that now exists. The effort to create an aesthetic wildlife habitat is visible all around and looks quite natural, though the destruction and subsequent reclamation are all at the hand of man.

NEARBY ATTRACTIONS

Boulder County Open Space: **bouldercounty.org/openspace**.

CHAUTAUQUA PARK: ROYAL ARCH

IN BRIEF

For the first-time visitor, as well as the native Boulderite, this is the perfect place to test your hiking mettle, with a serious elevation gain rewarded with a glimpse of the beautiful Chautauqua Park surroundings. Chautauqua Park lies on the southwestern edge of Boulder and is comprised of a park, cottages, auditorium, mountain park, and miles of mountain hiking trails.

DESCRIPTION

Start this hike by visiting the small ranger cottage off Bluebell Canyon Road and Baseline Road. Use the facilities, pick up a map, and go to the Chautauqua trailhead about 100 feet from the ranger's cabin. From the Chautauqua trailhead, take the Chautauqua Trail that ascends through Chautauqua Meadow at the base of the Flatirons.

The main trail is a loop that begins in a scenic meadow and then sharply ascends into the higher altitude forests. Royal Arch Trail begins where the loop trail returns down the mountain toward the trailhead. The base of the trail is well maintained, while upper portions of the trail are scattered with loose rock and steep rocky steps.

KEY AT-A-GLANCE INFORMATION

LENGTH: 3.46 miles
CONFIGURATION: Loop
DIFFICULTY: Moderate to difficult
SCENERY: Meadow, forest; views of University of Colorado, downtown Boulder; Flatirons (rock formations)
EXPOSURE: Sunny in meadow areas, increasingly shady at upper altitudes
TRAFFIC: Heavy
TRAIL SURFACE: Dirt, loose rocks, rocky at upper altitudes
HIKING TIME: 2.5 hours
SEASON: All year
ACCESS: Free
MAPS: USGS Eldorado Springs
FACILITIES: Restroom, ranger station
SPECIAL COMMENTS: Dogs must be leashed. Dogs may be off leash if the Voice and Sight Control tag is displayed. No overnight camping or backpacking. Climbers welcome. The trailhead is across the street from neighborhoods surrounding the CU campus. Erosion has taken a toll on this trail. On either side large rockslides can be seen. Biking is prohibited, and sections of seasonal wildlife closures (February 1–July 31) prevent a lot of out-of-bounds hiking.

Directions

From Denver, take I-25 north to US 36 to the Baseline Road exit and take a left turn, going west. Continue past the intersection of Broadway, and travel 1 mile to the entrance of Chautauqua Park, which is on the south side of the road. Pull directly into the large parking area at the trailhead, but if the lot is full (which it is most of the time), park along the south side of Baseline Road or along neighborhood streets.

GPS Trailhead Coordinates

UTM Zone (WGS84) 13S
Easting 0475895
Northing 4427448
Latitude N 39.996870°
Longitude W 105.282380°

N

0   0.15   0.3
mile

Flagstaff Rd.

Baseline Rd.

Gregory Canyon

P

Bluebell Canyon Rd.

Chautauqua Ranger Cottage

Chautauqua Trl.

Saddle Rock Trl.

Bluebell Mesa Trl.

Mesa Trl.

Bluebell Shelter

Enhanced Mesa Trl.

First Flatiron

Bluebell Canyon

Royal Arch Trl.

Mesa Trl.

T h e   F l a t i r o n s

Mesa Trl.

Skunk Canyon Trl.

Skunk Canyon

Royal Arch

8,500
8,000
7,500
7,000
6,500
6,000
5,500
5,000
4,500

FEET

1   2   3   3.46

MILES

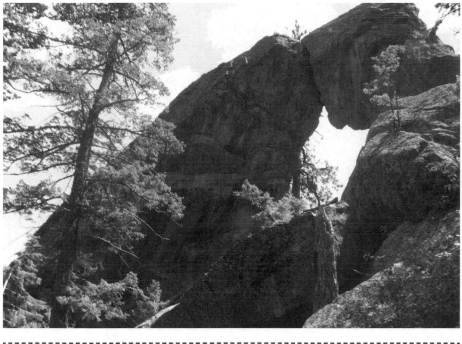

This hike's namesake—the Royal Arch—is magnificent up-close and personal. Right on the trail, it makes this a hike well worth the reward.

At 0.6 miles the Chautauqua Trail ends at a junction with the Ski Jump Trail and the Bluebell-Baird Trail. Continue straight until reaching the Bluebell Mesa Trail junction. At this point, the shade of the thickening pine trees offers a cool place for a short respite. Considering the sharp incline trail so far and what's ahead, a short rest and hydration break is a good idea.

Wide switchbacks continue up the side of the mountain before coming to another junction in the trail. A sign explains how to access the Ski Jump Trail on the right and Royal Arch Trail, Bluebell Mesa Trail, and Bluebell Shelter Trail on the left side of the trail. The Flatirons, colossal rock formations that jut up out of Chautauqua Park, are home to some of the best views of Boulder, Denver, and the Colorado Plains. There are five flatirons in Boulder: the northernmost flatiron being "one" and the southernmost flatiron being "five." Due to their sharp incline, the flatirons are highly exposed to the elements, leading to their accelerated erosion.

Take a left turn and spot a post without a sign at a fork in the trail. Turn right here at the fork onto the upper trail. Follow the third Flatiron access trail up a steep and winding path with many rocky steps. Find one of the many beautiful places to stop and take a quick respite. These areas allow for fantastic photo opportunities of the Flatirons and Boulder. Through the ascent, the path gradually thins and becomes increasingly difficult to navigate. Large rocks and loose gravel will make this part of the climb dicey. As the trail flattens slightly, another sign will offer access to the second and third Flatiron, as well as the Royal Arch Trail. Take the left-most path and ascend south along the Royal Arch Trail. At this point the trail becomes increasingly difficult. The trail switchbacks up the mountain with many rocks, both large and small, littering the path.

The noise from the more civilized portions of the trail will subside as the cool shade of the densely forested upper altitudes of the Flatirons provides some relief. The Royal Arch Trail is shaded most of the 0.8-mile ascent, but foliage is not an obstacle in most cases. Blueberries, wildflowers, and even the occasional cacti dot the less-steep side of the trail. Wildlife, however, is scarce, most certainly due to the trail's continual foot (and paw) traffic. After an arduous climb over the large rocky steps and steep ascent, the trail then leads to a false summit. While providing terrific views of Boulder, Longs Peak, the Indian Peaks, and the Flatirons, the summit gives the illusion of completion, only to dash those hopes as a sudden, short descent immediately turns into another steep climb to the Royal Arch. Keeping faith is important at this point. After another scramble up the rocky Flatiron, finally the Royal Arch comes into view.

The Royal Arch is an amazing natural structure and is a welcome sight to trail-weary travelers. Unfortunately, the Royal Arch does not offer very hospitable resting conditions, as the ground directly beneath the arch is rocky and uneven. The arch stands 20 feet above the ground and beautifully frames the Boulder valley below. The massive Flatirons can be seen to the north, where climbers can just barely be seen scaling the second Flatiron. The view is truly breathtaking, not that the hike wasn't.

Descending the Royal Arch Trail, while not as exhausting, is equally if not more difficult than the ascent. Back at the Royal Arch trailhead junction, take the Bluebell Road Trail down the mountain. Bluebell Shelter is located just below the trees as the rolling meadows reappear. The Bluebell Road Trail is a flat, well-established path with no obstacles, just an easy, gradual descent that allows for a nice cooldown before meeting up with the Chautauqua Trail again and back to the trailhead.

NEARBY ATTRACTIONS

Spend as much time as possible in the Chautauqua Park area while you are here. Rest in the large, shady park, which includes a playground. Check out the Chautauqua dining hall, community house, preservation office, lodges, and cottages. Maps for all of the Chautauqua buildings are available at the ranger station. For more information, visit the Web site for the City of Boulder Open Space and Mountain Parks, **bouldercounty.org/openspace,** or **chautauqua.com.**

ELDORADO CANYON: ELDORADO SPRINGS TRAIL

07

IN BRIEF

Eldorado Springs Trail is blessed with sunshine all year. Southern exposure makes this trail suitable for all seasons. Eldorado Canyon is world-famous for its rock climbing, and a multitude of climbers can be seen on the steep red rocks neighboring this trail. Occasionally, if the timing is right, you'll see trains traveling through the canyon. The trail can be a bit difficult but is broken up by flat sections that give it a more moderate rating.

DESCRIPTION

The trailhead is a short walk from the parking area. Cross the service road and begin the steep climb into North Draw. The switchbacks are well maintained, and steeper portions utilize man made staircases. Trail workers have taken obvious pains with signs and barriers to discourage cutting switchbacks. The trail is a well-worn dirt path lined with yucca plants, and most of it is very sunny and exposed.

   The man-made grade visible across the valley to the south is the railroad line that clings to the cliffs. SkiTrain and Amtrak use this line. At the top of the switchbacks, pass the technical climbing access signs to the Ricon Wall and others. You have great views to the north of technical climbing walls and Shirt Tail Peak.

KEY AT-A-GLANCE INFORMATION

LENGTH: 5.68 miles
CONFIGURATION: Out-and-back
DIFFICULTY: Moderate
SCENERY: Towering, sheer rock walls, views of railroad, pine trees, scattered forest, yucca
EXPOSURE: Sunny
TRAFFIC: Moderate
TRAIL SURFACE: Dirt, loose rocks
HIKING TIME: 4 hours
SEASON: All year
ACCESS: $3 walk-in, $6 October–April, $7 May–September, or annual state park pass; open sunrise to sunset
MAPS: USGS Eldorado Springs
FACILITIES: Restrooms, picnic tables
SPECIAL COMMENTS: Horses and dogs on leash are OK. No mountain bikes. Although this area is teeming with technical climbers, they usually park in a different area (on the road) and don't use this trail to get to their climbs. For technical rock climbing, Eldorado Canyon offers more than 500 different routes. Enthusiasts from all over the world come to Eldorado Canyon to enjoy some of the best climbing available.

Directions

From Denver, take I-25 north to US 36 west, toward Boulder. Exit at Louisville-Superior and turn left at the light. Take the first right onto CO 170 to Eldorado Canyon. Continue 7.4 miles through the canyon to the visitor center. After paying the park fee, travel 0.5 miles to the end of the road, where there is parking and picnic tables.

GPS Trailhead Coordinates

UTM Zone (WGS84) 13S
Easting   0474939
Northing   4419936
Latitude N 39.929161°
Longitude W 105.293290°

N

0   0.25   0.5
mile

South Boulder
Peak

BOULDER

MOUNTAIN

stone stairs

North Draw

Eldorado Springs Trl.

rockslide

Shirt Tail
Peak

saddle

Johnson Gulch

South Draw   South Boulder Creek

P

To Boulder

FEET

8,500
8,000
7,500
7,000
6,500
6,000
5,500
5,000
4,500

0.5   1   1.5   2   2.5   2.84

MILES

> Look up, look out, and look down in Eldorado Canyon. You don't want to miss a view.

The trail crosses a saddle, then travels into dense pine trees. Cross an old rockslide and continue up rock staircases. Here, the trail still provides views of the valley, Indian Peaks, and the Continental Divide. Signs dot the trail, which is worn and packed down, making it easy to follow. Cacti, yucca, and wildflowers grow on this hillside. The trail levels out, ascends once more, then levels out again, with good views of the area's sun-worshipping rock formations.

Descend from here, cutting across another massive old rockslide. Continue through a hillside of lodgepole and ponderosa pines, as well as juniper and pinon. Colorful boulders provide cover for some small springs. Travel past the boulders and rest, especially on hot days, since it is shaded and quite flat at this spot.

When we hiked, mountain lion tracks lined the trail for a few miles around this point, reminding us that it is always good to be aware of your surroundings.

From here, the trail curves, crosses over a ridge, and meanders through the same forest and boulders. Descend and cross a seasonal creek via tiny man-made bridges. Ascend more of the trail's characteristic switchbacks until the trees thin out. Here, you capture views of the plains to the left. Continue up the stone stairs. The rumbling sounds you may hear nearby are of the trains across the valley.

The trail opens into a modest meadow filled with yucca plants and ponderosa pines. The view is immense here, and you can see all the way to downtown Denver. South Boulder Peak looms high above as the trail cuts across the meadow and then descends fairly quickly into Walker Ranch. The Walker Ranch area and the back of Flagstaff Road can be seen to the north. The trail continues to descend and hikers may continue on, but the Eldorado Springs Trail unofficially ends here. Return the way you came.

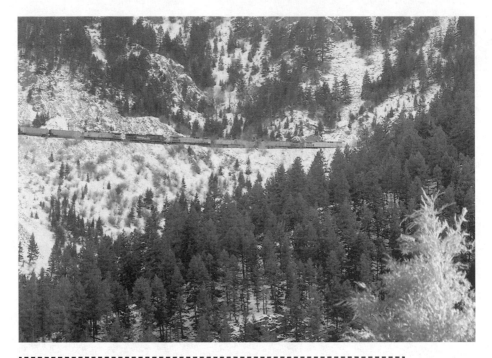

A train crossing, across the valley from the Eldorado Springs Trail. Hikers may hear the echo of the train whistle on railroad tracks cut into the mountain long ago.

NEARBY ATTRACTIONS

Walker Ranch Loop, Rattlesnake Gulch Trail, and Fowler Trail. For more information: **parks.state.co.us** and **bouldercounty.org/openspace.**

GREGORY CANYON: GREEN MOUNTAIN LOOP

IN BRIEF

This is a crowded "Boulder trail," but it's also a true gem and an excellent workout. Green Mountain Loop is comprised of four unique trails: Gregory Canyon Trail, Ranger Trail, E.M. Greenman Trail, and Saddle Rock Trail.

DESCRIPTION

Green Mountain Loop starts with the Gregory Canyon Trail, which begins from the right end of the Baird Park parking lot. Gregory Canyon Trail immediately intersects with Crown Rock Trail on the left. Head right, continuing on Gregory Canyon Trail toward a small creek, and then west along a ridge that crosses the creek and rises to the southwest. Watch for poison ivy along the trail, which is a former service road used for travel to gold mines near Central City. The trail is comprised of red dirt and loose rocks, and it ascends rather quickly in the beginning. We hiked in late fall, and slick, wet leaves were scattered on the trail. At this point, the well-maintained trail is only wide enough for one hiker at a time.

Cross an old wooden bridge that covers a small stream. As the terrain becomes more rugged and rocky, you face about 100 yards of semitechnical rock scrambling. No technical equipment is required, just steady footing.

KEY AT-A-GLANCE INFORMATION

LENGTH: 4.7 miles
CONFIGURATION: Loop
DIFFICULTY: Difficult
SCENERY: Creek, pine trees, historic buildings, rock formations
EXPOSURE: Mostly southern and shaded
TRAFFIC: Heavy with dogs and humans
TRAIL SURFACE: Dirt, loose rocks
HIKING TIME: 4 hours
SEASON: May–November; watch for early or late snows; check on closures February–July for raptor and bat habitats
ACCESS: $3 for parking (correct change only); open sunrise to sunset
MAPS: USGS Eldorado Springs, City of Boulder map at trailhead
FACILITIES: Dog refuse bags provided; restrooms, picnic table, and trash cans at trailhead and summit
SPECIAL COMMENTS: Unless your vehicle is registered in Boulder County and you're a Boulder County resident, you must pay $3 a day to park, or $15 a year. To avoid the parking fee, park at Chautauqua Park and walk to the trailhead. Dogs may be off leash if the Voice and Sight Control tag is displayed.

Directions

From Denver, take I-25 north to US 36 West. Exit west onto Baseline Road and take a left, going west to Chautauqua Park. Continue on Baseline, pass Chautauqua Park and the Flatirons, and turn left into the Gregory Canyon trailhead and Baird Park parking lot before the road takes a sharp right onto Flagstaff Road.

GPS Trailhead Coordinates

UTM Zone (WGS84) 13S
Easting   0475060
Northing   4427280
Latitude   N 39.995332°
Longitude   W 105.292155°

A view to the east in Gregory Canyon on the Green Mountain Loop.

The trail is now on a slight incline and continues uphill to more boulder fields. At a fork at the top of the hill, continue on the main path to the left. The trail merges with a fire road and continues south to Green Mountain Lodge.

This historic yet deserted building holds ghosts of miners, such as John Gregory, as well as pioneers and ranchers. Named after Gregory, the prospector who discovered the enormous Gregory lode behind Black Hawk, the Gregory Canyon Trail was originally built by settlers to provide wagon access to the gold fields near Black Hawk and Central City. According to historians, Gregory paid two miners the equivalent of $1.50 a day each to remove $1,000 of gold every week from the lode.

At the intersection of Flagstaff Road, Gregory Canyon Trail, Long Canyon Trail, and Ranger Trail, turn left onto Ranger Trail. Ranger Trail begins on the east side of the lodge and passes through ponderosa pine and Douglas fir forest to intersect with E.M. Greenman Trail.

Stay on Ranger Trail as it intersects with various Green Mountain trails coming in from the south. The last 0.8 miles of the Ranger Trail before the Green Mountain summit features loose rocks, a long ascent, and plenty of switchbacks. If hiking anytime after the first snowfall (as early as the first of September), watch for ice that collects on this southern-facing ridge. We hiked in November, and the last half mile was snow-packed and icy.

You'll find restrooms and picnic tables at the summit of Green Mountain. A summit marker and hiking register are at the top of a large boulder. The Colorado

Deserted Green Mountain Lodge provides a nice photo opportunity along the early part of Green Mountain Loop.

Hiking Club has installed a large bronze marker here that designates all of the major mountain peaks that can be seen from the summit. Some mountains are as far away as Rocky Mountain National Park and others as close as Indian Peaks Wilderness.

To start the descent, head back on E.M. Greenman Trail, opposite of the Ranger Trail. At the intersection of E.M. Greenman Trail and Saddle Rock Trail, take a right onto Saddle Rock Trail. Again, the downhill was steep and icy in early winter. The trail is much like the ascent, with switchbacks and steep rocks. To the west is the backside of the famous Boulder Flatiron rock formations and Chautauqua Park. Stay on Saddle Rock Trail as it veers to the left in the loop's last half mile. Saddle Rock Trail merges for a few yards with Gregory Canyon Trail, then ends back at the parking lot.

NEARBY ATTRACTIONS

Boulder trails, including the Flagstaff Mountain Loops and Chautauqua Loops. For more information, visit the Web site for the City of Boulder, Open Space and Mountain Parks: **bouldercounty.org/openspace.**

INDIAN PEAKS WILDERNESS: DEVIL'S THUMB LAKE

09

IN BRIEF

The hike to Devil's Thumb Lake is one of the classic hikes into Indian Peaks Wilderness. It is also one of the most popular, and often crowded, area hikes. This trail takes you into beautiful scenery that includes alpine meadows, mountain lakes, and views of snow-capped mountains. The hike is long and often wet but full of waterfalls in late spring and early summer. The trail crosses gently sloping terrain interspersed with steep stretches.

DESCRIPTION

Cross the creek via the wood bridge and come to a kiosk and the Hessie trailhead. Devil's Thumb Trail (#902) climbs steeply on an old road for 0.5 miles. The road is a very old, rough, four-wheel road that provides emergency Forest Service access. The Devil's Thumb Bypass turns right in 0.8 miles, just before the bridge. Either Devil's Thumb Trail or Devil's Thumb Bypass takes hikers to the same destination, and the distance is the same. At the bridge, near a thundering waterfall and a neighboring snowdrift, take a right onto Devil's Thumb Bypass. The bypass trail crosses

----

Directions ⟶

From Denver, take I-25 north to US 36 into Boulder. Turn left on Canyon Boulevard (CO 119), and travel all the way to Nederland (approximately 45 minutes). Stay on CO 119 going south out of Nederland for 0.5 miles. Turn right on CR 130, then follow signs to Eldora. Stay on CR 130 through Eldora and continue on dirt road. Bear left (staying on CR 130) at next fork and park here or drive 0.25 miles to Hessie trailhead up the dirt road. Note: Sometimes this road flows with runoff, since it is a cobblestone creek bed.

KEY AT-A-GLANCE INFORMATION

LENGTH: 11 miles

CONFIGURATION: Out-and-back

DIFFICULTY: Difficult

SCENERY: Dense forest, alpine tundra, high mountain peaks

EXPOSURE: Alternating sun and shade, high-altitude sunshine

TRAFFIC: Heavy, mostly on weekends

TRAIL SURFACE: Dirt, loose rocks, running water and wet areas, snowdrifts

HIKING TIME: 5.5 hours

SEASON: June–September (open all year)

ACCESS: Free, permits required for campers June–September 15; permits required for groups of 8 or more or organizational groups; group size limited to 12 people and pack stock combined; limited parking; open sunrise to sunset

MAPS: USGS East Portal and Nederland

FACILITIES: None

SPECIAL COMMENTS: Access to trailhead requires high-clearance vehicle and four-wheel drive; other cars park 0.25 miles before trailhead. No bikes or vehicles, dogs must be leashed, and special regulations for horses. In off-season, hikers can drive only to end of Eldora and ski or snowshoe in, then hike with winter gear.

GPS Trailhead Coordinates

UTM Zone (WGS84) 13S

Easting 0448675

Northing 4422620

Latitude N 39.952157°

Longitude W 105.600858°

N

0   0.5   1
mile

ROOSEVELT NATIONAL FOREST

To Nederland

CR 130

Hessie Trailhead

Lost Lake

Chittenden Mtn.

Lost Lake Trl.

Devil's Thumb Bypass

Devil's Thumb Trl.

Diamond Lake Trl.

CR 130

Jasper Creek

Woodland Lake Trl.

INDIAN PEAKS WILDERNESS

Woodland Mtn.

Middle Boulder Creek

King Lake Trl.

Diamond Lake

Woodland Mtn.

Jasper Lake

Devil's Thumb Trl.

Skyscraper Reservoir

Woodland Lake

Upper Diamond Lake

Devil's Thumb Lake

Devil's Thumb Pass

Continental Divide National Scenic Trl.

Devil's Thumb

ARAPAHO NATIONAL FOREST

CONTINENTAL DIVIDE

FEET

11,500
11,000
10,500
10,000
9,500
9,000
8,500
8,000
7,500

1   2   3   4   5   5.5

MILES

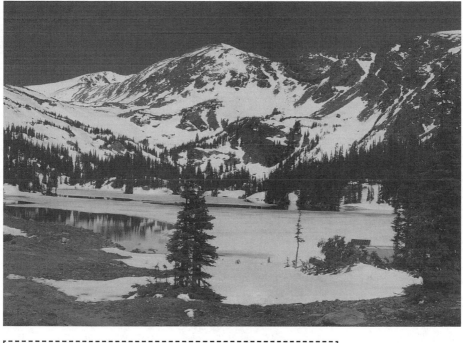

Devil's Thumb Lake at the base of Devil's Thumb is truly a sinful sight.

open meadows to the north of the creek. The main trail follows an old road along the south side of the creek, staying right past trail junctions with Lost Lake Trail, King Lake Trail, and Woodland Lake Trail. It is flooded most of the year and is best accessed in July.

The main trail bears to the right, goes uphill, and moves away from the creek a little bit. Social paths indicate that many hikers veer off of the main path to check out the waterfalls. The bypass trail is wet and has water running in places. As you continue to hike uphill, the trail opens into little meadows, with views of the Indian Peaks and the Continental Divide straight ahead. You now enter Indian Peaks Wilderness (marked with a sign) and travel a trail that is much easier to follow.

At the end of the meadows, the trail enters forest again. Continue gradually uphill through trees, and at the marked intersection, take a right back onto the main Devil's Thumb Trail. King Lake Trail and Woodland Lake Trail go left. The trail is now steep, ascending, and very rocky. The signs point out that this was once a mining road. Keep an eye out for when the mining road bears left uphill and the main trail goes to the right. You'll see a little sign that points hikers to the right. The trail is wider here, and the sound of waterfalls reminds you that you're never far from the main creek.

Eventually the trail comes back and runs parallel to the same mining access road. Cross the road and stay on the trail with a stream to the right. We hiked in mid-June, and snowbanks dominated the trail. Here it is steep and rocky, and

A waterfall along Devil's Thumb Trail. One of the many water features you will see—some quiet, some thunderous.

the elevation climbs. You're encouraged to travel up and over the snowbanks in the trail even if they are rather large. Continue up the rock stairs on the other side of the creek.

Eventually, the trail joins up again with the old mining road. Don't be discouraged by the steepness of the trail—it levels out soon. Traverse the ridge, which is an old four-wheeling road that was cut into a shelf road. The shelf road continues across an old rockslide. At this point, you're in a big mountain basin surrounded by a cirque of high peaks.

Continue straight past the turnoff to Diamond Lake Trail and travel 0.6 miles to Jasper Lake, which is surrounded on three sides by trees and a steep ridgeline. Here you cross a spillway with a bridge traveling through shallow water. Often a social plank is placed across the spillway 100 yards downstream. The trail continues another mile over a small ridge, north of a pond, and up a slope to Devil's Thumb Lake. It lies directly below the vertical wall of Devil's Thumb. Rest before you turn around and head back to the trailhead.

NEARBY ATTRACTIONS

Hessie trailhead is also the trailhead for the Continental Divide and Devil's Thumb Pass, and other Boulder Ranger District Trails (Lost Lake Trail #813, King Lake Trail #901, and Woodland Lake Trail #811). For more information, visit the Web site for the USDA Forest Service, Arapaho and Roosevelt National Forest, Pawnee National Grassland: **fs.fed.us** (reference Devil's Thumb Trail #902).

INDIAN PEAKS WILDERNESS: GLACIER RIM TRAIL

IN BRIEF

Arapaho Glacier is the most southern glacier in the Rocky Mountains, and it is melting. This trail takes you to the glacier along a high and exposed route that earns its place among the longest and most difficult in this book. Not much is left of the glacier, which is surrounded by high mountain peaks and alpine tundra, but its destination is a reward and a good turn-around point. An alternate access leads to the glacier overlook, but this one is a better work-out, is more scenic, and is less used.

DESCRIPTION

The Glacier Rim Trail (#905) trailhead is well marked and is just after the one-way sign near the end of the road. Hike past the wilderness sign that marks the Indian Peaks Wilderness boundary and continue straight. Pass a barbed-wire fence to your right and a sign indicating City of Boulder Watershed. This area is the source for most of Boulder's drinking water and is heavily patrolled. Public access is prohibited.

The first several miles of this hike follow the watershed boundary, so please stay on the trail. The high elevation causes a shortness of

KEY AT-A-GLANCE INFORMATION

LENGTH: 12.2 miles

CONFIGURATION: Out-and-back

DIFFICULTY: Difficult

SCENERY: Alpine tundra, high mountain peaks; views toward Boulder

EXPOSURE: Shaded for first few miles, then exposed due to high altitude

TRAFFIC: Light

TRAIL SURFACE: Hard-packed dirt, extremely rocky

HIKING TIME: 6.5 hours

SEASON: June–September (open all year)

ACCESS: Free, permits required for campers June–September 15; permits required for groups of 8 or more or organizational groups; group size limited to 12 people and pack stock combined; open sunrise to sunset

MAPS: USGS Monarch Lake and Ward

FACILITIES: Restroom

SPECIAL COMMENTS: Special regulations for horses, no bikes or vehicles, and dogs must be leashed. Hikers can only drive to gate where road forks in off-season and ski or snowshoe in, then hike with winter gear. Trail is not well marked and hard to follow in bad weather. Exposed to sun, wind, hailstorms, and blizzards, even mid-summer. Go equipped accordingly.

Directions

From Denver, take I-25 north to US 36 into Boulder. Turn left on Canyon Boulevard (CO 119) and travel all the way to Nederland (approximately 45 minutes). At the traffic circle, go north on CO 72 for 7.5 miles, until you see a sign for University of Colorado Mountain Research Station. Turn left there on FR 298 (CR 116), go 1 mile, bear left on the same road, and travel 4.5 miles until the end of the road. Two trailheads are next to one other: The first one is Glacier Rim Trail.

GPS Trailhead Coordinates

UTM Zone (WGS84)   13T

Easting   0451240

Northing   4428880

Latitude   N 40.008708°

Longitude   W 105.571301"

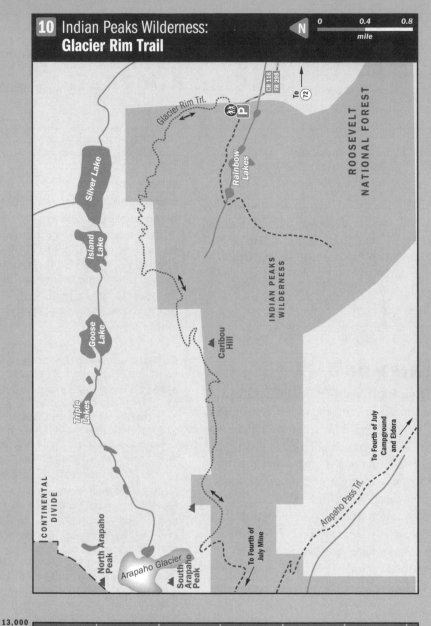

10 Indian Peaks Wilderness:
Glacier Rim Trail

N

0   0.4   0.8
mile

CR 116
FR 298

To 72

ROOSEVELT
NATIONAL FOREST

Glacier Rim Trl.

P

Silver Lake

Rainbow Lakes

Island Lake

INDIAN PEAKS
WILDERNESS

Goose Lake

Caribou Hill

Triple Lakes

To Fourth of July
Campground
and Eldora

CONTINENTAL DIVIDE

Arapaho Pass Trl.

North Arapaho Peak

Arapaho Glacier

South Arapaho Peak

To Fourth of
July Mine

FEET						
13,000						
12,500						
12,000						
11,500						
11,000						
10,500						
10,000						
9,500						
9,000						
	1	2	3	4	5	6.1

MILES

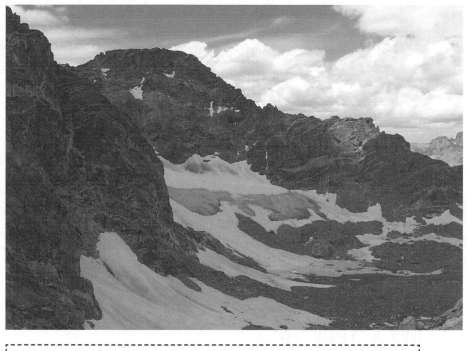

True to its name, Glacier Rim Trail offers views of Arapaho Glacier and South Arapaho Peak.

breath. Even at the trailhead, this is evident in the short stature of the vegetation.

Travel through occasional switchbacks as the trail gets steeper and climbs at each turn. The trees end abruptly, and the rest of the hike is left very exposed. After reaching timberline, you're treated to incredible views into the heart of Indian Peaks Wilderness. Glance over your right shoulder and look for Silver Lake. As the trail goes straight southwest, up Caribou Hill, it switches back to the right, around the north to the top. Across the valley are views of Niwot Ridge. From here you can see the University of Colorado Mountain Research Station.

Notice the tree line is higher across the valley due to the southern exposure and constant sunshine. A switchback high up on the northern slope will take you through jumbled rocks. The last switchback (for a while) puts you on a long southwest traverse.

Pass the top of Caribou Hill to the left and set your sights on the next ridge. The Corona Bowl of Eldora Ski Area, along with Barker Reservoir, will now be visible, and the town of Nederland can be seen off to the left. A new group of mountain peaks comes into view to the southwest, and just as it does, the trail switchbacks going the other way, to the north.

Traverse the south slope and ascend. To the left are some of the long, narrow glacial valleys left from when the Rocky Mountains were created. Several hikes in this book are in that direction, including Devil's Thumb Lake and Heart Lake. James Peak is directly south. This traverse includes a welcome, mild descent.

After the downhill, continue due west across the next hillside. Pass an extremely weathered sign, right in the middle of the hillside, indicating 1 mile to Arapaho Glacier. The traverse remains level for a while, crossing an extremely rocky slope. Enjoy the level and slight downhill grade because the trail starts climbing again.

At the beginning of the climb, glance over your left shoulder to see the Fourth of July trailhead and, in a few moments, South Arapaho Peak and its pyramid shape straight in front. A trail on the left that goes down to Arapaho Pass Trail and Fourth of July Trail is in fact a steeper, faster way down in case of an emergency, but there is no telephone until the town of Eldora. That trail continues by way of the Arapaho Pass Trail as it goes west, over the Continental Divide toward Grand Valley and Winter Park.

Reach the Arapaho Glacier overlook in the shadow of South Arapaho Peak. From this point, ambitious hikers can continue as the trail goes up the south side of the peak with a little scrambling required. Otherwise, turn around from here and head back the 6.1 miles to the car.

Note that hikers with two cars can leave one at Fourth of July trailhead above Eldora and do a shuttle hike.

NEARBY ATTRACTIONS

Rainbow Lakes Trail #918, Arapaho Pass Trail #904, and other Indian Peaks Wilderness hikes: **fs.fed.us/r2/arnf.**

INDIAN PEAKS WILDERNESS: MOUNT AUDUBON

11

IN BRIEF

Hikers reach Mount Audubon by a strenuous march straight up to 13,000 feet from 10,000 feet. The hike's trailhead may be enough beautiful alpine scenery for some, but the higher panoramic alpine views and alpine lakes are quite rewarding. Those who take this challenge will be above tree line for most of the hike and exposed to alpine elements and tundra.

DESCRIPTION

Start from the north corner of the parking lot at the Beaver Creek trailhead. The trail is well maintained and well marked, and it proceeds directly into a subalpine evergreen forest. Enjoy the gentle grade and the shade for a short time, since the trail will climb, become very steep, and eventually emerge from the trees, becoming totally exposed for the remainder of the hike.

Views to the east stretch across the plains. You can also see Brainard Lake, Long Lake, Niwot Ridge, and the nearby Indian Peaks. Follow the trail as it traverses across the eastern slope.

Directions ────────────────────▶

From Denver, take I-25 north to US 36 into Boulder. Turn left on Canyon Boulevard (CO 119) and travel all the way to Nederland (approximately 45 minutes). Go north on CO 72 to the small town of Ward. Look for the signs that indicate a left turn to Brainard Lake Recreation Area, and turn left onto CR 102. Go toward Brainard Lake; come to a gate where the $7 fee is collected. The road becomes one-way and travels counterclockwise around the lake. Follow the signs to the Mitchell Lake Area and turn right. Park at the Mitchell Lake trailhead parking area.

(i) KEY AT-A-GLANCE INFORMATION

LENGTH: 8.4 miles

CONFIGURATION: Out-and-back

DIFFICULTY: Difficult

SCENERY: High mountain views, including Indian Peaks

EXPOSURE: Above tree line, exposed to wind, sun, and lightning storms

TRAFFIC: Moderate (can be heavy, especially on weekends)

TRAIL SURFACE: Dirt, very rocky, loose trail

HIKING TIME: 4.5 hours

SEASON: June–September (open all year)

ACCESS: $9 for five-day pass per vehicle, $45 season pass; open sunrise to sunset

MAPS: USGS Ward

FACILITIES: Emergency telephone, restrooms, picnic areas, campgrounds

SPECIAL COMMENTS: No bikes or vehicles, camping limitations with permits required for overnight visits, and dogs must be leashed. The last section of this hike is above timberline and exposed to violent lightning. Time hikes for early morning with a minimum noon summit goal. In the off-season, hikers must park near the highway and ski or snowshoe in, then use snowshoes for the hike.

GPS Trailhead Coordinates

UTM Zone (WGS84) 13T

Easting 0450510

Northing 4436930

Latitude N 40.081190°

Longitude W 105.580468°

N

0   0.25   0.5
mile

R O O S E V E L T
N A T I O N A L   F O R E S T

Waldrop North Trl.

To Nederland

BRAINARD LAKE
RECREATION AREA

Brainard Lake

Beaver Creek Trl.

Beaver Creek Trl.

Mt. Audubon Trl.

Mitchell Lake Trl.

I N D I A N   P E A K S
W I L D E R N E S S

Mitchell Lake

Mt. Audubon

Blue Lake

FEET

13,500
13,000
12,500
12,000
11,500
11,000
10,500
10,000
9,500

1   2   3   4   4.2

MILES

The alpine views and alpine lakes are awe-inspiring on Mount Audubon Trail.

At 1.3 miles, the Beaver Creek Trail goes right down to Coney Flats Road. Veer left on Mount Audubon Trail. Views to the north open up to Longs Peak and Mount Meeker. You'll face Mount Audubon at this point, and it tends to loom in the distance as the climb continues. The trees disappear as the trail cuts over a small stream and across an alpine meadow to a snowfield. Even into June and July, the trail will climb toward the snowfield, taking a sharp right and climbing through a boulder field to a flat ridge.

A direct headwind is normal for the remainder of the hike, and the real huffing and puffing begins after a few switchbacks. At 3.5 miles, the trail bears left up a steep and rocky portion before it eventually comes to a flat square spot in the tundra and disappears. Go left and scramble up the rock face.

Follow the cairns and take the main route to the summit. You'll think you can see the peak, but it is not visible and still requires approximately 20 minutes of steep scrambling from the bottom of the rock face. Stop and take a breath, since 13,000 feet has thin air. Keep scrambling up the rock face as it does finally level off, signaling the summit of Mount Audubon. Rest, enjoy the summit, and turn around to head back to the trailhead.

NEARBY ATTRACTIONS

Beaver Creek Trail #911, Mitchell and Blue Lakes trails #912, and Pawnee Pass Trail: fs.fed.us/r2/arnf.

12 JAMES PEAK WILDERNESS: HEART LAKE

KEY AT-A-GLANCE INFORMATION

LENGTH: 7.96 miles

CONFIGURATION: Out-and-back

DIFFICULTY: Difficult

SCENERY: Dense forest, alpine tundra, high mountain peaks

EXPOSURE: Shaded until tree line, high-altitude sunshine

TRAFFIC: Moderate

TRAIL SURFACE: Dirt, loose rocks, tree roots

HIKING TIME: 4.5 hours

SEASON: June–September (open all year)

ACCESS: Free; open sunrise to sunset

MAPS: USGS East Portal and Empire

FACILITIES: None

SPECIAL COMMENTS: Hikers must cross a creek multiple times, and it is likely that your feet will get wet, so be sure to wear the appropriate foot gear. Dogs are allowed and recommended to be leashed, but it's not mandatory. The regulations are less strict than in other wilderness areas, but still prohibit bikes, strollers, or anything wheeled, except for aiding a disabled person. Horses and camping are allowed.

GPS Trailhead Coordinates

UTM Zone (WGS84) 13S

Easting   0444985

Northing   4416955

Latitude   N 39.900887°

Longitude W 105.643576°

IN BRIEF

Several hikes in the book, such as South Boulder Creek, follow South Boulder Creek in lower elevations. This hike goes to Rogers Pass Lake and Heart Lake, the source of South Boulder Creek. The hike travels through cool, dense spruce and fir forest, leading up into a beautiful alpine basin ringed with high mountain peaks. Hikers frustrated with parking in nearby Indian Peaks Wilderness will have an easy time here. This trail is less crowded than its neighbors.

DESCRIPTION

Follow the small signs in the northwest area of the parking lot pointing to the trail. Start out on South Boulder Creek Trail #900. The trail immediately enters aspen and pine forest that is lush in late summer and dotted with wildflowers. A five-minute walk takes you to a kiosk with trail information.

The trail immediately passes the railroad facilities at the east portal of the Moffat Tunnel. The big buildings primarily house

Directions

From Denver, take I-25 north to US 36 into Boulder. Turn left on Canyon Boulevard (CO 119), and travel all the way to Nederland (approximately 45 minutes). Stay on CO 119 going south out of Nederland for 5 miles into Rollinsville. Take a right onto CR 16 (Forest Road 149). Go 7 miles to where CR 16 (FR 149) technically ends, but the road continues on. Go straight here and follow sign directions to East Portal. Be extremely careful of the two railroad crossings on the road. This is a heavily used railroad line, including simultaneous trains traveling in different directions. Some automobiles have to wait a long time while trains are being switched in this valley.

To Nederland

South Boulder Creek

P

East Portal

Nebraska Hill

Union Pacific and Burlington Northern Santa Fe Railroads

Moffat Tunnel

Forest Lakes Trl.

South Boulder Creek Trl.

Crater Lakes Trl.

Crater Lakes

South Boulder Creek

Clayton Lake

Heart Lake

Rogers Pass Lake

Rogers Pass

CONTINENTAL DIVIDE

Iceberg Lakes

FEET

11,500
11,000
10,500
10,000
9,500
9,000
8,500
8,000
7,500

1   2   3   3.98

MILES

The east portal of Moffat Tunnel, one of the longest railroad tunnels in the country.

ventilators. Don't be alarmed if the ventilator fans come on when you're walking by. At 6.2 miles, this is one of the longest railroad tunnels in the United States, and the large ventilators are for the diesel fumes.

Railroad buffs may want to also take a drive up Rollins Pass. The original railroad route was constructed over the top of the Continental Divide. Rollins Pass is a right turn about 1.5 miles before the trailhead.

Parallel to the railroad tunnel is a water tunnel operated by the Denver Water Board that brings water from the western side of the Continental Divide to the Denver metropolitan area. Follow the trail as it curves right near an old cabin. South Boulder Creek rushes down on the left. You'll parallel this creek for most of the hike. After crossing Arapaho Creek on a wooden bridge, look up to the right and glimpse a beautiful, cascading waterfall.

A stroll on the paths to the left takes hikers into heavily forested campsites. Hike straight through the cool, dense evergreen forest along a very gradual uphill. As the trail becomes rockier and the forest becomes dense, you'll pass many trees draped with lichen and mosses.

At the intersection with Forest Lakes Trail, continue straight up via a switch-back. The trail now opens up to high mountain meadows with remnants of old cabins. You'll gain substantial elevation above South Boulder Creek and can look down and see waterfalls that feed into the creek.

Sturdy bridges built in the 1990s have eliminated many wet creek crossings, but at this point, you should still be ready to walk on a very wet trail. Continue to travel uphill. An occasional trail goes off the left near the waterfalls and the creek, but more waterfalls are coming up, and you might as well stay on the trail.

Views from the trail will make your heart pitter-patter as it pumps along on Heart Lake Trail.

Begin consistent switchbacks away from the creek. At this point, the trail becomes narrow, steep, and rocky, and is marked by an occasional red dot on the trees. Continue straight at the intersection with Crater Lakes Trail. Walk across the boards that have been laid to help navigate difficult sections. Due to snow-drifts and water in springtime, many trails meander around this area, so pay attention to the red dots and the trail. It's always apparent within a minute or two if you're on the main trail or not.

If you veer off the trail and get lost, just remember to go back toward South Boulder Creek. For the first 3 miles of this hike, the trail does not stray too far from the creek. Cross a small log bridge over a side creek, then immediately cross another small log bridge over the main South Boulder Creek. Continue hiking along the south side of the creek. After a short while, you switchback to the left, away from the creek. Here, in late spring or early summer, you'll encounter snowdrifts. The Forest Service requires everyone to hike through the snowdrifts and water so the trail is not further eroded.

After about 15 minutes, cross the next bridge and go through a site often used for camping. Walk across the wet area on the other side and continue. This is the last bridge, and the remainder of the trail is extremely wet. As hikers approach 11,000 feet, the trees start to thin, and most people will have significant shortness of breath. The trees open up here, and hikers are rewarded by stunning alpine scenery; Haystack Mountain and James Peak are to the left. Take a right at the fork to Heart Lake and the trail will continue uphill to the namesake lake. At Heart Lake, turn around and trace the route back to the trailhead. Going left will take hikers to Rogers Pass Lake and the Continental Divide.

13   WALKER RANCH: MEYERS HOMESTEAD TRAIL

KEY AT-A-GLANCE INFORMATION

LENGTH: 5 miles

CONFIGURATION: Out-and-back

DIFFICULTY: Moderate

SCENERY: Open meadow, old homestead, stream; scattered aspen trees, willow trees, and ponderosa pines

EXPOSURE: Partial shade, mostly exposed

TRAFFIC: Heavy

TRAIL SURFACE: Dirt, sandy

HIKING TIME: 2.5 hours

SEASON: All year

ACCESS: Free; open sunrise to sunset

MAPS: USGS Eldorado Springs

FACILITIES: Picnic areas, restrooms

SPECIAL COMMENTS: Leash law for dogs is strictly enforced; tickets are issued for noncompliance. Boulder County Open Space provides loaner leashes at the trailhead. Self-serve fee stations are all the way up Flagstaff Road, but no fee is required at Walker Ranch. No motorized vehicles. Meyers Homestead Trail can be crowded with mountain bike traffic, but not as crowded as neighboring Walker Ranch Loop.

IN BRIEF

Walker Ranch has two popular hikes, and Meyers Homestead Trail is definitely the laid-back sibling of the Walker Ranch Loop. This peaceful hike travels along a spacious fire road through aspens, meadows, and ponderosas. It even travels back in time, passing by an old homestead. A jogging stroller glides right along and gives Mom and Dad quite a workout, thanks to a gradual climb that gets the blood flowing.

DESCRIPTION

Leave the parking area and head toward the trailhead, which is marked by a kiosk. The trail descends slowly and empties into an open meadow before descending again and emptying into a smaller meadow. To the left is the old Meyers Homestead and the trail's namesake. Colorado homesteaders staked their claim here in the late 1800s. This high-country valley would have looked much the same, yet would have been considered quite rugged since most Colorado settlements were not yet thriving.

A small stream follows along the left of the trail, which begins a gentle ascent. You may see deer that find shelter and forage in the willow and aspen trees that border the stream. A hill on the right is covered with

GPS Trailhead Coordinates

UTM Zone (WGS84) 13S

Easting   0471130

Northing   4422910

Latitude   N 39.955835°

Longitude   W 105.337998°

Directions

From Denver, take I-25 north to US 36 to Baseline Road in Boulder; go left. Take Baseline Road west until it turns into Flagstaff Road. Travel 7.5 miles total from US 36 to Walker Ranch trailhead on the right.

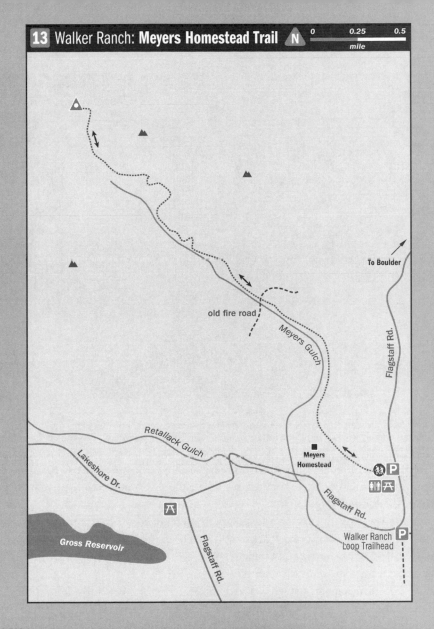

N

0   0.25   0.5

mile

To Boulder

old fire road

Meyers Gulch

Flagstaff Rd.

Retallack Gulch

Lakeshore Dr.

Meyers
Homestead

Flagstaff Rd.

Walker Ranch
Loop Trailhead

Gross Reservoir

Flagstaff Rd.

8,500

8,000

7,500

7,000

6,500

6,000

5,500

5,000

4,500

FEET

0.5   1   1.5   2   2.52

MILES

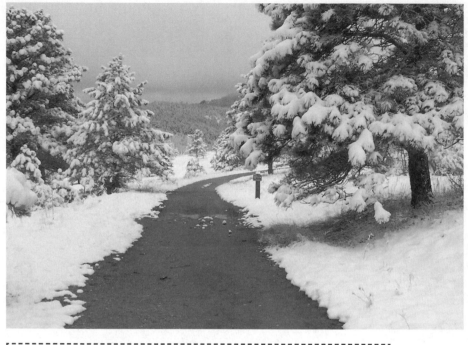

Trees bear the weight of a new snow along the Meyers Homestead Trail. The path has remarkably kept clear—just a little wet—and attests to the warmth of the earth.

large boulders, sparse ponderosa pines, and wildflowers. Cross a culvert and continue climbing. After 1 mile the trail reaches an intersection with an old fire road. Continue straight.

Follow the trail as it roller-coasters up and down the gully that has been carved by the stream. Loose rocks and tree roots begin to appear on the trail, but it is still spacious and sandy. Smaller streams and tributaries meet up with the larger stream that follows the trail.

The trail becomes steeper and exposed. Pass a steep hillside and an aspen forest, then enter into a large meadow 2 miles into the hike. This broad, green meadow is filled with wildflowers and wild grasses. To the left is another small stream lined with aspens and willows. The trail climbs through the meadow and reaches a crest in the hill. From here, you can look north and east to Boulder.

Continue as the trail curves west into the rocks and trees. Reach a saddle that signifies the end of the trail. The overlook at trail's end points to views of Sugarloaf Mountain and the Indian Peaks and farther to views of Longs Peak. Turn around here and retrace the route back to the trailhead.

NEARBY ATTRACTIONS

All Walker Ranch Trails and Eldorado Canyon Trails: City of Boulder Open Space and Mountain Parks. Visit **bouldercounty.org/openspace**.

Denver (Including Foothills and Mountains)

N

| 0 | 5 | 10 |

miles

DENVER
(INCLUDING FOOTHILLS AND MOUNTAINS)

14 ALDERFER THREE SISTERS OPEN SPACE PARK: PONDEROSA SISTERS LOOP

ⓘ KEY AT-A-GLANCE INFORMATION

LENGTH: 3 miles

CONFIGURATION: Double loop

DIFFICULTY: Moderate

SCENERY: Open, marshy meadow; boulder fields, forest

EXPOSURE: Exposed in meadow, shady in other areas

TRAFFIC: Moderate

TRAIL SURFACE: Dirt, loose rocks

HIKING TIME: 1.75 hours

SEASON: All year

ACCESS: Free; open 1 hour before sunrise to 1 hour after sunset

MAPS: USGS Evergreen, Conifer

FACILITIES: Picnic table, restrooms

SPECIAL COMMENTS: Dogs must be leashed at all times. Collection of wildflowers or other natural resources is prohibited. Bears and mountain lions have been seen on this trail, and users must report any sightings to Open Space Rangers or call Jefferson County Natural Resources at (303) 271-5993.

IN BRIEF

Alderfer Three Sisters Open Space Park boasts 770 acres of open land. Ever since Evergreen was settled, the four rock formations called Three Sisters and Brother have been landmarks, providing views of the Bear Creek Basin and Mount Evans. More than 10 miles of trail lead hikers around the Three Sisters and up to Brother. Ponderosa Sisters Loop is a great way to take a cursory look at this mountain park.

DESCRIPTION

Head out of the parking lot and take a right onto Bluebird Meadow Trail as it curves eastward past an old barn by the trailhead. The trail travels through open meadow, which is grassy and marshlike in early summer. Reach the Bluebird Meadow and Silver Fox trail crossing and turn left onto Silver Fox Trail.

Pass the Homestead Trail crossing, but continue straight on Silver Fox. As the trail curves east through the meadow, you see your first views of the Three Sisters. Pass another Homestead Trail crossing and continue straight on Silver Fox.

At the intersection of Ponderosa and Silver Fox trails, go left on Ponderosa Trail, leaving the meadow for ponderosa pine and woodland forest. Travel 0.2 miles to the intersection of

GPS Trailhead Coordinates

UTM Zone (WGS84)   13S

Easting   0469150

Northing   4385750

Latitude   N 39.620955°

Longitude   W 105.359432°

Directions ⟶

From Denver, take I-70 west to Evergreen Parkway (CO 74). Go left, traveling south on CO 74 to Evergreen. Turn right onto CO 73, then turn right at the stoplight onto Buffalo Park Road. Take Buffalo Park Road 2.3 miles to the trailhead and parking lot on the right, just before reaching Le Masters Road.

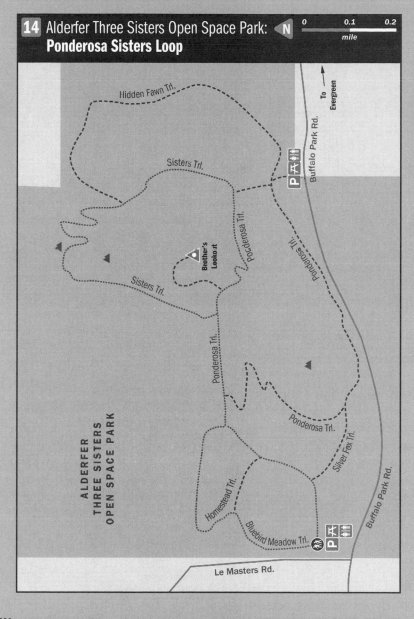

N

| 0 | 0.1 | 0.2 |

mile

To
Evergreen

Hidden Fawn Trl.

Sisters Trl.

Buffalo Park Rd.

P

Ponderosa Trl.

Brother's
Lookout

Ponderosa Trl.

Sisters Trl.

Ponderosa Trl.

**ALDERFER
THREE SISTERS
OPEN SPACE PARK**

Ponderosa Trl.

Silver Fox Trl.

Homestead Trl.

Buffalo Park Rd.

Bluebird Meadow Trl.

P

Le Masters Rd.

8,500		
8,000		
7,500		
7,000		
6,500		
6,000		
5,500		
5,000		
4,500		

FEET

0.5   1   1.5   2   2.5   3

MILES

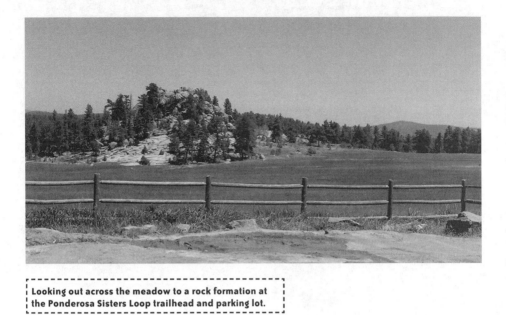

Looking out across the meadow to a rock formation at
the Ponderosa Sisters Loop trailhead and parking lot.

Ponderosa and Sisters trails. Take a left on Sisters Trail (full of loose rocks, sand, and exposed tree roots). The next 1.3 miles are the most difficult of this hike.

Cut straight across the hillside and prepare for a series of switchbacks that travel between the second and third sisters. Reach a saddle in the trail after the long ascent and look out toward Evergreen Lake on the left and Evergreen High School on the right. After cresting the hill, the hike is a steady and forgiving downhill. Sisters Trail intersects with Hidden Fawn Trail; continue straight on Sisters Trail. The trail is flanked by quaking aspen trees and low, thick brush.

At the intersection of Ponderosa Trail and Sisters Trail, go straight onto Ponderosa Trail and climb three distinct switchbacks. The Brother and a turnoff to Brother's Lookout are to the right, but stay straight on Ponderosa Trail. Pass a familiar intersection with Sisters Trail and Ponderosa Trail after completing one loop, then continue straight on Ponderosa Trail, retracing old trail. At the intersection of Silver Fox Trail and Homestead Trail, take a right on Silver Fox Trail and then an immediate right on Homestead Trail. To complete the second loop, follow Homestead Trail around the north side of the rock formation. Reach the intersection of Homestead Trail and Bluebird Meadow Trail and take a right on Bluebird Meadow Trail. Follow it back into the meadow, where the trail is comprised of wooden walkways in the wettest portions. Come out at the far end of the parking lot, or continue around the split-rail fence to the trailhead.

NEARBY ATTRACTIONS

Alderfer Three Sisters Open Space Park has 14 hiking trails with 10 miles of hiking; for more information, visit the Web site for Jefferson County Open Space at **jeffco.us/openspace.**

BARR LAKE STATE PARK: LAKE PERIMETER TRAIL

 15

IN BRIEF

The Lake Perimeter Trail at Barr Lake offers a rare opportunity to explore a major prairie reservoir in Colorado. The lake is lined with cottonwoods, marshes, and aquatic plants. Its southern half has been designated as a wildlife refuge to shelter animals and birds, including the 350 species of birds that have been spotted here.

DESCRIPTION

Turn right out of the parking lot and the area around the Barr Lake Nature Center. The trail begins 100 yards from the lake, and it was muddy when we hiked in late fall. Cottonwood trees provide some shade in the morning and complete shade in the afternoon. Along with cottonwood trees, irrigation ditches line the trail, and two such ditches are found to the left and right of the trailhead. The trail starts counterclockwise from the nature center, and the mile markers are for those traveling the other direction on the Pioneer Trail to the wildlife observation station and gazebo on the lake.

You see houses at the beginning of the trail, but they disappear as prairie meadows and cottonwood trees take over all line of sight. Early in the trail, hikers may encounter horseback riders and mountain bikers. Continue to a

KEY AT-A-GLANCE INFORMATION

LENGTH: 9.2 miles

CONFIGURATION: Loop

DIFFICULTY: Easy

SCENERY: Lake, prairie, cottonwoods, dam, and irrigation ditches

EXPOSURE: Shaded in cottonwoods, open and exposed in other areas

TRAFFIC: Mild

TRAIL SURFACE: Paved, dirt

HIKING TIME: 4.5 hours

SEASON: All year, muddy in shoulder seasons

ACCESS: $5 or Colorado State Park Pass, open 5 a.m.–10 p.m.; Crest Trail is closed Wednesdays and Saturdays October–February.

MAPS: USGS Brighton, Mile High Lakes

FACILITIES: Pay phone, restrooms, nature center, ranger station; picnic areas with tables and grills

SPECIAL COMMENTS: No pets. No swimming or wading; boating is permitted. Collecting living or dead plants, wood, or animals (wildlife and insects) is prohibited. Fishing and waterfowl hunting is permitted. Sturdy shoes are recommended. Irrigation companies use the trail; hikers are asked to yield right of way to their personnel and equipment.

Directions ————————→

From Denver, take I-76 northeast to the Bromley Lane exit. Take a left, going east on Picadilly Road, then another left, going south to the park entrance. Follow the paved road from the ranger station to the nature center and the trailhead.

GPS Trailhead Coordinates

UTM Zone (WGS84)   13S

Easting   0521280

Northing   4420610

Latitude   N 39.935337°

Longitude   W 104.750937°

Lake Perimeter Trail offers incredible views across Barr Lake.

parking area (for boat-ramp users) and a gate; cross the paved road and go through the gate on the other side. The dam comes into view across the lake. Continue around to the east. At the northeast corner of the lake is a big sign that says the lake is 8.8 miles around. Go left here and follow the dirt road that travels to the back of the dam.

At this point, the grass-covered dam is to the left and elevated about 10 feet above the trail. On the right is an irrigated field, but no other signs of civilization are visible here.

Pass mile marker 7 and continue to pass these mile markers going backward. Due to the unique views and ease of the trail, they seem to go by rather quickly. Cross an irrigation ditch where the water exits the reservoir. Numbered blinds for bird hunting line the trail.

Continue left up the dam on the Barr Lake Crest Trail. The hill is steep for 100 yards, but it deposits hikers directly onto the top of the dam. The trails run parallel at this point, one on the top and the other on the bottom to the right. From here you see views of the mountains, including, most prominently, Longs Peak.

The upper and lower trails merge at the northwest part of the dam. Pass the Bruderlin Stone House and the Rocky Mountain Bird Observatory office. Veer left, continue along the lake, and travel alongside I-76 with its traffic noise. A gate and private property are to the left, and the trail veers to the right of that, with barbed wire on both sides. The western side of the lake is the wildlife refuge, which does not have as much traffic as the other side. The trail, which is double-track dirt with low grasses on either side, runs about 0.25 miles from the lake. Go through an opening in the fence, cross the road, and enter the gate on the other side. Continue on an old doubletrack along train tracks to the right.

While the trail is flat, various thorns have collected and are quite dense here. Continue along the lake and take a left before the next gate. Bear left down a small hill toward the lake. Continue straight behind a dozen homes, some with horses in back. The trail takes a sharp right after the last house.

Quite a few marshes are along the trail, and to the right is a cattle pasture and a bald eagle nesting area. Warning signs advise all trail users to stay out.

Take a left at an intersection of the trail and the main road; do not go straight on the main road. The trail is now a well-maintained gravel walking path. This area of the reservoir is a little more active, with more bald eagles and more signs of human life. Cross the bridge over a large irrigation ditch and continue as the trail rejoins a service road. Go left; pass the gazebo and boardwalk on the lake used for wildlife viewing. Pass another observation area and head back to the parking lot.

NEARBY ATTRACTIONS

The Gazebo Trail (or Pioneer Trail) is a shorter (3 miles) trail at Barr Lake. For more information: **parks.state.co.us.**

BEAR CREEK LAKE PARK: BEAR CREEK TRAIL

16

IN BRIEF

The 2,500 acres of prime real estate that make up Bear Creek Lake Park have all the makings of an urban hideaway. Located in Lakewood, just southwest of Denver, Bear Creek Lake Park sits at the base of the foothills. Its grassy dam catches the waters of both Bear and Turkey creeks. Bear Creek Trail follows Bear Creek and winds through giant cottonwoods and across arid prairie without any telltale urban signs. Remote sounds from nearby roads are the only hint that civilization is close by.

DESCRIPTION

Leave the parking area and cross Morrison Road to the start of Bear Creek Trail, which is concrete here and perpendicular to Morrison Road. Immediately take a left, start through the canopied river basin, and walk parallel to Bear Creek. Walk through the entrance of Bear Creek Lake Park and pass the ranger station. Since you parked outside the park and foot traffic is not regulated, you don't have to pay.

Follow the entrance road until it intersects with a trail right before Skunk Hollow. Go left and begin to head toward Bear Creek Reservoir. There is no sign here, but the trail is obvious.

KEY AT-A-GLANCE INFORMATION

LENGTH: 4.42 miles
CONFIGURATION: Balloon
DIFFICULTY: Easy
SCENERY: Bear Creek, Bear Creek Reservoir, plains, riparian ecosystem
EXPOSURE: Mostly shaded
TRAFFIC: Heavy in spots
TRAIL SURFACE: Hard-packed dirt, paved in portions
HIKING TIME: 2 hours
SEASON: All year
ACCESS: Free;
May–Labor Day, 6 a.m.–10 p.m.;
April and October, 7 a.m.–8 p.m.;
November–March, 8 a.m.–6 p.m.
MAPS: USGS Morrison
FACILITIES: Visitor center, marina, 50 picnic sites, restrooms, 4 reservable park shelters, 50 campsites
SPECIAL COMMENTS: This trail starts outside the Bear Creek Lake Park, but if hikers choose to start inside the park, entrance fees are $4 for a general daily pass or $40 for an annual pass. Dogs must be leashed and may not swim in the creeks or lakes within the park.

Directions

From Denver, take C 470 south to the Morrison Road/CO 8 exit. Park across from the Conoco Break Place just after exiting C 470.

GPS Trailhead Coordinates

UTM Zone (WGS84)   13S
Easting   0484330
Northing   4389040
Latitude   N 39.651011°
Longitude   W 105.182650°

Reach the intersection of Owl Trail and Visitors Center Trail and take a left onto Owl Trail. Pass the Owl Trail marking posts with the owl silhouettes and numbers.

Travel along the river and stay on the south bank, even though bridges cross Bear Creek via side trails. A horse trail, the Fitness Loop, and the Owl Trail all converge at a crossroads. Continue straight and pass a trail that goes up over the ridge.

Bear Creek Reservoir comes into view as the trail begins to veer away from the roar of Bear Creek. The terrain is still river basin, but the trail is wider and flanked by tall grasses. The dirt is less compact and loosens up into a sandlike consistency. Travel up a hill, leaving the river completely, and enter a semiarid landscape. Go around a bend and come out to a newly constructed picnic shelter with deluxe beach volleyball and horseshoes. This area, called Pelican Point, is the 2-mile mark and sits at the base of the Bear Creek Reservoir Dam and its small overflow lake. The trail passes Pelican Point and then makes a large U-turn to the right and continues, passing a horse arena.

After you cross a small bridge, the trail parallels a road for a short while. At 2.85 miles and an obvious fork in the trail, take a right turn back toward the creek bed. Follow the pedestrian-marked trail and take a left. Hit the 3-mile point and begin to backtrack on the familiar Owl Trail. Go straight across the road to the Skunk Hollow picnic area. Do not turn right and go back to the ranger station. Go through the parking lot, pass a covered picnic site, and get back on the trail behind the picnic grills. Reach the concrete Bear Creek Trail, take a right, and cross a bridge. Immediately take a left, head back to the start of Bear Creek Trail, cross Morrison Road, and go back to the car.

NEARBY ATTRACTIONS

Bear Creek Lake Park has 15.7 miles of trails. The Mount Carbon Loop is the park's longest hike at 6.9 miles. Visit the city of Lakewood's Web site for more information: **lakewood.org**.

17 DEER CREEK OPEN SPACE PARK: MEADOWLARK PLYMOUTH CREEK LOOP

KEY AT-A-GLANCE INFORMATION

LENGTH: 2.5 miles

CONFIGURATION: Loop

DIFFICULTY: Moderate

SCENERY: Foothills, meadows, scrubby hillside, forest, stream; views of Denver and Deer Creek Valley

EXPOSURE: Exposed on Meadowlark Trail and last portion of Plymouth Creek; lush sections on rest of Plymouth Creek

TRAFFIC: Heavy

TRAIL SURFACE: Smooth and hard-packed dirt; loose rocks

HIKING TIME: 1.5 hours

SEASON: All year

ACCESS: Free; open sunrise to sunset

MAPS: USGS Indian Hills

FACILITIES: Restrooms (handicap accessible), covered picnic tables, pay phone, drinking water

SPECIAL COMMENTS: Dogs are allowed but must be leashed. Dog refuse pickup bags provided at trailhead. This Jefferson County trail is hiker only on the Meadowlark Trail portion.

IN BRIEF

Deer Creek Canyon has a good mix and 12.2 miles of multiuse trails, but the hiker-only options are what really attract pedestrians. This is a popular location, close to Denver with access all year, and it can be quite crowded with mountain bikes. No bikes are allowed on the Meadowlark Trail, where hikers can enjoy a gradual climb, sunny exposure, southern views of Denver, and views of the Deer Creek Valley.

DESCRIPTION

Leave the abundant facilities at the trailhead and go right. Take an immediate left onto Meadowlark Trail, and follow the HIKER ONLY signs. Pass through Rattlesnake Gulch and its sage scrub and prairie grasses as the trail begins to climb at a steady 10 percent grade. Look east and northeast at new luxury homes and a Lockheed Martin campus.

Travel through two switchbacks and the trail opens to views west, up Deer Creek Canyon. Looking west, it is eerie to think that Colorado's most famous cannibal, Alfred Packard, lived and worked his last years in this area.

The trail has ascended for 1 mile and now roller-coasters up and down with flat

----

GPS Trailhead Coordinates

UTM Zone (WGS84) 13S

Easting 0486840

Northing 4376880

Latitude N 39.541487°

Longitude W 105.153152°

Directions

From Denver, take C 470 south 6.7 miles to Kipling Parkway; exit south. Go right on West Ute Avenue, and turn right again on Deer Creek Canyon Road. Follow Deer Creek Canyon Road west 2.7 miles to Grizzly Road. Turn left on Grizzly Road, and follow it 0.4 miles to the park entrance on the right.

N

0   0.1   0.2
mile

Deer Creek Canyon Rd.

Deer Creek

Rattlesnake Gulch

To
Denver

P

Meadowlark Trl.

Grizzly Rd.

Meadowlark Trl.

Plymouth Creek Loop

Bill Couch
Mtn.

Plymouth Creek Loop

Plymouth Creek

Plymouth Mountain Trl.

8,500

8,000

7,500

7,000

6,500

6,000

5,500

5,000

4,500

FEET

0.5   1   1.5   2   2.5

MILES

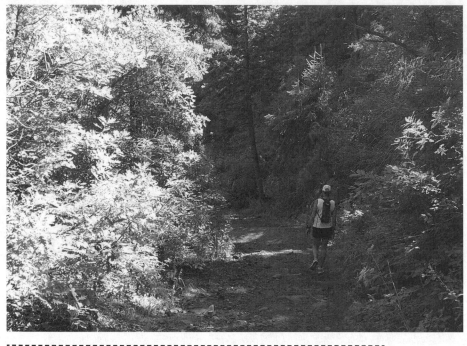

A summer hiker getting a nice, shady respite on Meadowlark Plymouth Creek Loop.

sections in between. The trail is cut into the hillside and comes close to the edge many times, so steady footing is required.

Continue onto the backside of the scrubby hillside, and the trail again reaches the east-facing slopes. There, it crosses the southeast face of the mountainside with views of the southern plains, downtown Denver, and the hogback.

Traverse two ravines and descend to a bridge in a lush, pine-shaded valley. At the intersections of Meadowlark Trail and Plymouth Creek Loop, take a left and begin a steady descent. The trail is wide and steep with loose rocks as it follows Plymouth Creek. Although mountain bikers are permitted here, they must travel up this steep, technical section and prove no space challenge to hikers.

The trail skirts the south side of the ravine as you cross through three switchbacks and head northeast. The trail travels up and down along the edge of the hillside, eventually leading back to the southern side of the trailhead.

NEARBY ATTRACTIONS

South Valley Park, 6.9 miles of trails (Swallow Trail is hiker only): **jeffco.us/ openspace.**

DENVER: WASHINGTON PARK 18

IN BRIEF

Washington Park, known as Wash Park to locals, is an urban haven for fitness enthusiasts. Along with its proximity in the South Denver Park District, it is home to amazing facilities, National Historic Landmark park buildings, and an easy hike. Take in this hike on an early weekend morning and then treat yourself to a stroll through the beautiful neighborhoods that surround Wash Park.

DESCRIPTION

Leave your parking space and find a spot on the Wash Park Trail just before Kentucky Avenue. Travel north along the crushed-granite path that outlines Wash Park or travel along the shoulder of the asphalt road that follows along the Wash Park Trail. The trail is well maintained and surrounded by manicured grass. Continue to walk through the large cottonwood and maple trees, and pass the maintenance facility at 820 South Humble Street. Pass older park buildings to the left and coveted bungalow homes to the right. An old wagon with big red wheels sits along the trail, hinting at Denver's pioneer beginnings. Stay on the path around the park as it alternates between asphalt and crushed gravel.

Pass the Wash Park recreation building on the left and soon start a counterclockwise trip

KEY AT-A-GLANCE INFORMATION

LENGTH: 2 miles

CONFIGURATION: Loop

DIFFICULTY: Easy

SCENERY: Urban park with mature trees, lakes

EXPOSURE: Mostly shaded

TRAFFIC: Heavy

TRAIL SURFACE: Dirt, concrete, grass, and asphalt

HIKING TIME: 45 minutes

SEASON: All year

ACCESS: Free; open 6 a.m.–11 p.m.

MAPS: USGS Englewood

FACILITIES: Restrooms, picnic facilities, tennis courts, basketball courts, recreation center, pay phone, playgrounds, lawn-bowling park, boating, fitness course, fishing, soccer field, boathouse pavilion, youth fishing pond, flower gardens, and croquet park

SPECIAL COMMENTS: Dogs must be leashed, and you must pick up all waste. Watch out for vehicle traffic. Be aware of other dogs. Pit bulls are not allowed in Denver city limits. Washington Park hosts many public events, so check a Denver newspaper or Web site before heading out, which will save the headache of hiking during a crowded festival.

Directions

From Denver, take I-25 south to the South University Boulevard exit and go left, traveling north through the Washington Park neighborhood. Turn left (west) on Mississippi Avenue. Turn right on Franklin Street, which is the east boundary of Washington Park, and park in this vicinity. The starting point is two blocks north, near Kentucky Avenue, which is perpendicular to South Franklin Street.

GPS Trailhead Coordinates

UTM Zone (WGS84) 13S

Easting 0502650

Northing 4394210

Latitude N 39.697734°

Longitude W 104.969091°

18 Denver: Washington Park

N 0   0.1   0.2
mile

E. Virginia St.

S. Marion Pkwy.

Lily Pond

E. Center Ave.

P Doschappell Bathhouse

Smith Lake

E. Exposition Ave.

Boathouse Pavilion

P

Washington Park Recreation Center

P

Smith Ditch

E. Ohio Ave.

S. Humboldt St.

S. Downing St.

WASHINGTON PARK

S. Franklin St.

E. Kentucky Ave.

lawn

E. Tennessee Ave.

P

Smith Ditch

E. Mississippi Ave.

Grassmere Lake

LAWN BOWLING PARK

S. Gilpin St.

E. Arizona Ave.

Tennis Courts

E. Louisiana Ave.

25

(Right column duplicates street names: E. Virginia St., E. Center Ave., E. Exposition Ave., E. Ohio Ave., E. Kentucky Ave., E. Tennessee Ave., E. Mississippi Ave., E. Arizona Ave., E. Louisiana Ave.)

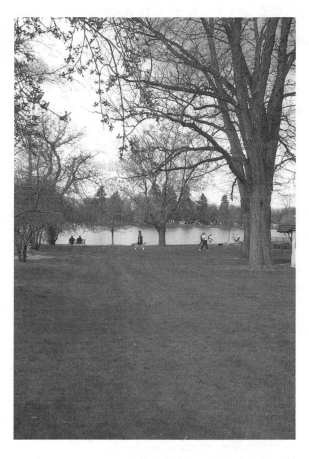

Weekend warriors, busy along the ponds, grass, and trails in Washington Park.

around Smith Lake. You'll find an old boathouse pavilion on the south end of the lake. Continue around the lake. Across the street from the northeast side is a youth fishing pond (Lily Pond). Local duck populations call both the lake and the pond home. Continue through a shaded canopy provided by large pines. Hikers can find old stone picnic tables and barbecue pits here.

On the right, you pass a large apartment building and a memorial statue that is set back from the trail. The trail begins to curve to the left once you pass another entrance to Wash Park at Virginia Street. Its surface is more consistently dirt and gravel as hikers pass the Doschappell Bathhouse, which is home to Volunteers for Outdoor Colorado. Pass the intersection and the Wash Park entrance of Exposition Avenue and Downing Street.

On the right is one of 54 flower gardens within the park's 165 acres. Spring color begins with iris and peonies. Near the large garden is a 1926 replica of the Martha Washington garden at Mt. Vernon, Virginia.

Follow the bend as it curves left to a playground and large parking area. Cross over a small irrigation canal that is part of the Smith Ditch Historic District. Continue and pass horseshoe, tennis, and basketball courts on the left.

Soon the trail begins to border larger Grasmere Lake. Continue along its perimeter in a counterclockwise motion. To your immediate left, a boardwalk extends over the lake. At the south end of the lake, you'll find tennis courts, bathrooms, and a pay phone. Pass over the Smith Ditch once more as you approach the east side of Grasmere Lake. Cross Mississippi Avenue and venture back into the park.

NEARBY ATTRACTIONS

Denver parks, shopping, restaurants, and attractions: **denvergov.org**; Washington Park Recreation Center: (303) 698-4962.

19 ELK MEADOW OPEN SPACE PARK: SLEEPY S LOOP

KEY AT-A-GLANCE INFORMATION

LENGTH: 2.5 miles

CONFIGURATION: Balloon

DIFFICULTY: Moderate

SCENERY: Forest, boulder field, mountain view

EXPOSURE: Partly shaded

TRAFFIC: Moderate

TRAIL SURFACE: Dirt, loose rocks

HIKING TIME: 1.5 hours

SEASON: All year

ACCESS: Free; open 1 hour before sunrise to 1 hour after sunset

MAPS: USGS Evergreen

FACILITIES: Picnic tables, restrooms

SPECIAL COMMENTS: Dogs must be leashed at all times. Across Stagecoach Boulevard, you'll find an off-leash dog park with a 0.3-mile hiking trail. Collection of wildflowers or other natural resources is prohibited. Bears and mountain lions have been spotted on this trail, and users must report any sightings to Open Space Rangers or call Jefferson County Open Space at (303) 271-5925.

IN BRIEF

As the name suggests, Elk Meadow's trail system is home to elk and deer. Hiking the Sleepy S Loop almost guarantees deer sightings. Perhaps it's the secluded pine forest or the meadow and mountain views that attract the deer and sometimes the elk. Either way, it's a beautiful place to call home and a beautiful place for a moderate hike.

DESCRIPTION

Start in the parking lot and go right onto Meadow View Trail as it climbs gently to the northeast. The wide dirt trail is well maintained and flanked on both sides by erosion-control railway ties. Pass a picnic table directly to the right. A staircase to the left leads to a hidden picnic area.

Keep moving on Meadow View Trail and pass a restroom on the left. These facilities are a small hike from the trailhead.

The trail ascends and starts a roller coaster before leveling out. After 0.3 miles, take a right on the Sleepy S Trail as it intersects with Meadow View Trail. Start a gradual descent and pass covered picnic tables and benches scattered about.

The trail takes a large curve to the left and continues to descend before it levels out a

GPS Trailhead Coordinates

UTM Zone (WGS84) 13S

Easting 0468570

Northing 4389240

Latitude N 39.652379°

Longitude W 105.366355°

Directions

From Denver, take I-70 west to Evergreen Parkway (CO 74). Go left, traveling south on CO 74 to Stagecoach Boulevard. Turn right, and travel 1.25 miles to the south parking lot.

N

0   0.15   0.3

mile

Too Long Trl.

Meadow View Trl.

Palmer's Pause Trl.

Evergreen Pkwy.

Founders Trl.

74

**ELK MEADOW
OPEN SPACE PARK**

Elk Ridge Trl.

Bergen Peak Trl.

Sleepy S Trl.

Meadow View Trl.

Meadow View Trl.

South
Trailhead

Stagecoach Blvd.

To 74
and Evergreen

FEET

8,500
8,000
7,500
7,000
6,500
6,000
5,500
5,000
4,500

0.5   1   1.5   2   2.5

MILES

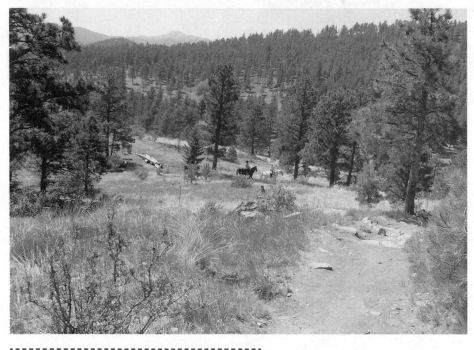

Equestrians share the road along the Sleepy S Loop.

little and begins to climb again. Pass through shady ponderosa pine trees. Once the trail reaches the grassland and the views, you will see the intersection of Sleepy S Trail and Elk Ridge Trail. Take a left onto Elk Ridge Trail, which ascends gradually into ponderosa pine tree stands, switchbacks a few times, and continues to climb. Continue up, up, up at a steady pace for 0.5 miles.

Reach the intersection of Meadow View Trail and Elk Ridge Trail. Go left onto Meadow View Trail and immediately pass the Bergen Peak Trail trailhead. The trail descends, sometimes steeply, through the tall, widely spaced ponderosa pine trees. Reach the intersection of Meadow View Trail and Sleepy S Trail and take a right, heading back to the trailhead.

NEARBY ATTRACTIONS

Elk Meadow Open Space Park has seven hiking trails with 13 miles of hiking. For more information, visit the Web site for Jefferson County Open Space: **jeffco.us/ openspace.**

EVERGREEN: EVERGREEN LAKE 20

IN BRIEF

Evergreen Lake reflects the beauty of this mountain town: a sparkling creek, pine trees, sunshine, and a calm, serene demeanor. A small dam with cascading water sits at the opposite end of the lake house. The hike around Evergreen Lake is a splendid respite from the Denver bustle.

DESCRIPTION

Head toward the lake house, which is visible from the entrance. At the lake house, take a left to a boardwalk that covers a large, marshy area. This is the start of the Evergreen Lake Trail clockwise around the lake. Continue on the boardwalk and go over the bridge that crosses Bear Creek as the creek enters Evergreen Lake.

Cross another feeder bridge and take a sharp right before the road. Walk on the trail, which travels along the road on the left and the lake on the right. Reach the dam and you can see downtown Evergreen in the distance. Walk down the stairs to the spillway, just below the dam. A high-altitude garden is planted here. Cross a long bridge that spans Bear Creek, walk in front of the dam's waterfall, and head up the stairs on the left. Now the lake is on your right, and the mountainside and mountain residences are on your left. To the left are staircases built into the rocks that lead to a lake lookout.

Directions

From Denver, take I-70 west to Evergreen Parkway (CO 74). Go left, traveling south on CO 74 to Evergreen. Turn right on Upper Bear Creek Road, and take it around to the entrance of Evergreen Lake.

KEY AT-A-GLANCE INFORMATION

LENGTH: 1.28 miles
CONFIGURATION: Loop
DIFFICULTY: Easy
SCENERY: Mountain lake
EXPOSURE: Partly shaded
TRAFFIC: Moderate
TRAIL SURFACE: Dirt, paved, bridges
HIKING TIME: 1 hour
SEASON: All year
ACCESS: Free; open 5 a.m.–11 p.m.
MAPS: USGS Evergreen
FACILITIES: Lake house, boat rentals, ice-skate rental, restrooms, picnic tables, grills
SPECIAL COMMENTS: The beautiful log lake house is open to the public and available to rent for special events. Call (720) 880-1300 for facility information, or visit evergreenrecreation.com. The fishing pier is handicap-accessible. Ice-skating season lasts from mid-December to mid-March, weather permitting. Summer activities include non-motorized boating and outdoor concerts. The southwest side of Evergreen Lake on Upper Bear Creek Road is an Evergreen Golf Public Course; call the pro shop for more information: (303) 674-6351.

GPS Trailhead Coordinates

UTM Zone (WGS84) 13S
Easting 0471550
Northing 4386680
Latitude N 39.629418°
Longitude W 105.331510°

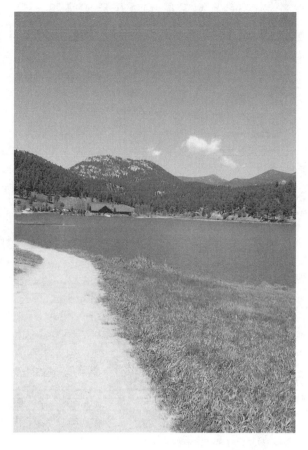

Evergreen Lake is seen from all angles on this hike. The magic of the mountain water only leaves the view for a short while.

Stay on the lower portion of the trail, and do not head up to the road. Get on a wooden boardwalk as it crisscrosses in and out over the lake. Cross another bridge and come around to the Evergreen Meadow side. Switchback as the trail ascends onto an upper portion of the trail. On this hillside, you'll overlook the lake and the old ice-skating shelter. Do not go to the shelter. Instead, go right and head back to the lake house and the end of the trail.

NEARBY ATTRACTIONS

Denver Mountain Parks manages many of Evergreen's parks. See its Web site for more information: **denvergov.org**.

Most of Evergreen's open space parks and hiking trails are managed by Jefferson County Open Space: **jeffco.us/openspace**.

21 GOLDEN GATE CANYON STATE PARK: MOUNTAIN LION TRAIL

KEY AT-A-GLANCE INFORMATION

LENGTH: 6.36 miles

CONFIGURATION: Loop

DIFFICULTY: Difficult

SCENERY: Green mountain meadows, lush aspen groves, pine-covered hills, freshwater creeks, views of Denver

EXPOSURE: Mostly shaded

TRAFFIC: Mild

TRAIL SURFACE: Hard-packed dirt, loose rocks

HIKING TIME: 4 hours

SEASON: May–October

ACCESS: $6 for the day or $60 annual state parks pass; open sunrise to sunset

MAPS: USGS Ralston Buttes; maps at visitor center

FACILITIES: Outhouse; no facilities at this trailhead, but restrooms, picnic spots, and campsites in the park

SPECIAL COMMENTS: Hikers must cross a creek multiple times, so wear appropriate footgear. This is a multiple-use trail for hikers, bikers, and equestrians. Leashed dogs are permitted. Fishing is allowed in any stream or pond except the visitor center show pond. For scheduling information for weddings at Panorama Point Scenic Overlook, call the park office at (303) 582-3707.

- -

GPS Trailhead Coordinates

UTM Zone (WGS84) 13S

Easting   0469210

Northing   4411010

Latitude   N 39.848551°

Longitude W 105.359915°

IN BRIEF

Seldom visited, Golden Gate Canyon State Park is just outside of Golden and 25 miles west of Denver. The park offers a few large loop trails, and rangers at the visitor center recommend this one. Mountain Lion Trail is a rugged mountain trail with great views that offers hikers plenty of solitude.

DESCRIPTION

Head east out of the parking lot and get onto the Mountain Lion Trail. The singletrack trail immediately starts an uphill climb. A stream flows downward on the left. Hikers are transported from the start to the feel of the backcountry. The trail is hard-packed, rocky, and only wide enough for a single hiker.

The trail cuts across a hillside and makes a large, arched switchback. Trails in this park are named after animals and have an accompanying symbol on signage. The Mountain Lion Trail's symbol is a mountain lion paw print.

Cross a gully with a seasonal stream, and continue across the hillside. The area is lightly wooded with tall evergreen trees. Views of evergreens extend to the surrounding hillsides.

- -

Directions

From Denver, take I-70 west to CO 58 traveling toward Golden. Turn right off of CO 58 onto CO 93, and after 2 miles, turn left on Golden Gate Canyon Road at the Golden Gate Canyon State Park sign. The road winds 13 miles to the visitor center. Stop here to buy your park pass for the day. Take a right out of the visitor center parking lot and continue on Ralston Creek Road, which actually leaves the state park for 1 mile before reentering. Continue 3 miles; pass a number of trailheads until you see the Nott Creek sign. Turn left here, and drive to the Mountain Lion trailhead parking lot.

N

0   0.2   0.4
mile

To old quarry

Mountain Lion Trl.

GOLDEN GATE
CANYON
STATE PARK

Deer Creek

service
roads

Mountain Lion Trl.

Nott Creek

Mountain Lion Trl.

P

Ralston Creek Rd.

Burro Trl.

Burro Trl.

Burro Trl.

Burro Trl.

To visitor center
and Golden

Windy
Peak

To City Lights Ridge

Forgotten
Valley

Mountain Lion Trl.

Buffalo Trl.

A snow-covered bridge in a winter wonderland on Mountain Lion Trail.

Come to an intersection with a doubletrack service road and take a right. Continue across an open hillside. A service road veers to the left, but the Mountain Lion Trail continues straight. It is very well marked, and an intersection such as this one is signed with the mountain lion paw.

The trail descends slightly into ponderosa pines. Continue down into the valley, where you can hear the sounds of gurgling Deer Creek. Here the trail becomes dense with mature pine trees. When you cross Deer Creek by traversing a wooden footbridge, look for mining gear and a large, old mining boiler in the water. Take a left after the bridge and head toward Windy Peak. To the right is a former quarry. The trail here is a narrow, rocky singletrack that parallels the creek.

Cross Deer Creek again and enter a rocky area that leads away from the creek. Here you'll find a well-marked backpacking campsite. It is a premier campsite and worth making a mental note for your next trip to Golden Gate Canyon. More of these campsites come into view, and each one is reached by crossing a private little bridge that straddles the creek. Take the trail across Deer Creek on another small wooden footbridge. A smaller side trail goes to a sleeping shelter.

Here, the rocky, wooded trail begins to ascend. Continue straight at the intersection of Burro Trail and Mountain Lion Trail, and follow the signs to Windy Peak. The trail is still narrow, flanked by thick brush, pine trees, and willow trees. For the next half mile, continue in this heavy growth along the creek. Follow a number of bridges that crisscross over the water for 2 miles. The terrain opens up a bit and becomes less overgrown. The trail is still near Deer Creek in the bottom

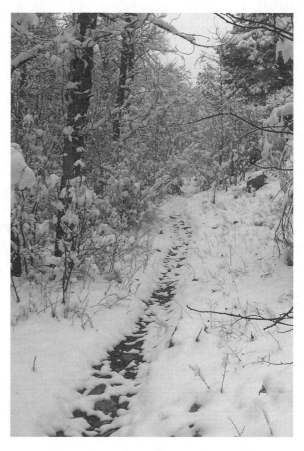

More winter beauty along a snowy Mountain Lion Trail.

of a gully. As it continues its gradual ascent, the hillside becomes rocky, with views of boulder fields.

Enter a lodgepole pine forest and follow a couple of long, steep switchbacks, going left just before an old barbed-wire fence. The trail continues across the hillside, ascending steep switchbacks. Pass another intersection with Burro Trail that cuts off to Windy Peak. Hike to the top of a ridge, go over, and drop down to a severe descent. Descend an extremely steep hill before the trail levels out and cuts across a hill overlooking an early settlement now called Forgotten Valley. The trail switchbacks and descends quickly, going to the bottom of this valley and joining up with Nott Creek. It is easy hiking from here, down an old, abandoned service road. The trail quickly turns back into a singletrack with small rocks and gravel and ascends for five minutes.

Continue straight past the intersection with the Buffalo Trail, which turns right to Rifleman Phillips Group Campground. Pass an intersection to City Lights Ridge. Merge with the Burro Trail, and jog to the left on Mountain Lion Trail to go back to the Nott Creek trailhead.

The trail levels out and goes across the top of a ridge before the trail drops down. As you approach Ralston Creek Road, take a sharp left and descend toward the access road to the parking lot. The trail parallels the access road and comes out in the far corner of the parking lot where you started.

NEARBY ATTRACTIONS

Try the 11 additional trails in Golden Gate Canyon State Park. See the Colorado State Parks Web site for more information: **parks.state.co.us.**

22 LAKEWOOD: GREEN MOUNTAIN AND HAYDEN TRAIL LOOP

KEY AT-A-GLANCE INFORMATION

LENGTH: 3.3 miles

CONFIGURATION: Loop

DIFFICULTY: Difficult

SCENERY: Open fields, views of metro Denver

EXPOSURE: No shade

TRAFFIC: Heavy

TRAIL SURFACE: Dirt, loose rocks

HIKING TIME: 2.5 hours

SEASON: All year

ACCESS: Free; open 5 a.m.–10 p.m.

MAPS: USGS Morrison

FACILITIES: Restrooms

SPECIAL COMMENTS: Dogs are allowed but must be leashed at all times. Mountain bikers and equestrians use this trail, so be cautious.

IN BRIEF

The slopes and summit of Green Mountain are in Lakewood's second-largest park—William Frederick Hayden Park—covering 2,400 acres of open space. The steep terrain here includes a challenging system of trails and great views of the city. Some locals come every day to run the trail featured here. One time up the slope and hikers will either love it or regret it.

DESCRIPTION

Start in the parking lot, where you can see Green Mountain, and head right. Go straight up the steep hillside. After a half mile of exertion, reach a fork in the trail and go left to continue the ascent. Proceed up and across the hillside and travel through open meadow and seasonal wildflowers.

At the intersection of Green Mountain Trail and an established cut-through trail, continue straight on Green Mountain Trail. As you catch your breath, glance at views of metro Denver, including downtown Denver and the southwest Denver area. Bordered only by short brush, the trail is well maintained, considering its exposure and heavy use.

At the 1-mile point, the trail begins to level out and ascend gradually. Pass a large radio tower on the right. You see mountain

GPS Trailhead Coordinates

UTM Zone (WGS84) 13S

Easting 0486940

Northing 4393150

Latitude N 39.688087°

Longitude W 105.152309°

Directions

From Denver, take I-70 west to C 470 south. Exit at West Alameda Parkway (CO 26), and turn left onto West Alameda Parkway. The trailhead is on the left at West Florida Drive.

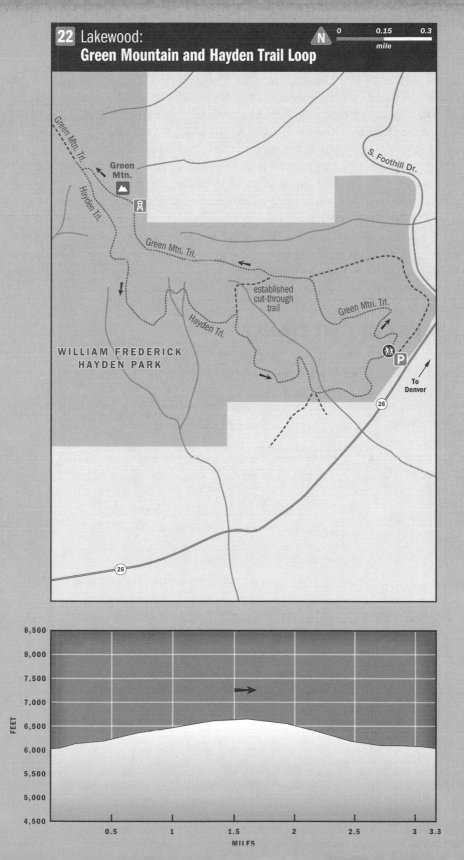

N

0   0.15   0.3
mile

Green Mtn. Trl.

Hayden Trl.

S. Foothill Dr.

Green
Mtn.

Green Mtn. Trl.

established
cut-through
trail

Green Mtn. Trl.

Hayden Trl.

WILLIAM FREDERICK
HAYDEN PARK

P

To
Denver

26

26

8,500

8,000

7,500

7,000

6,500

6,000

5,500

5,000

4,500

FEET

0.5   1   1.5   2   2.5   3   3.3

MILES

views to the left and Denver over your shoulder to the right. Turn left at the tower and travel on a path wide enough for two hikers to walk side by side.

Reach an intersection of Green Mountain Trail and Hayden Trail at 1.33 miles, and take a sharp left. Red Rocks and Dinosaur Ridge are visible to the right. The trail begins a slight descent, cutting into the hillside with gradual switchbacks. As it continues to descend and come around to the western side of the mountain, the trail opens up to views of the hogback. Any roaring engines are the sounds from cars and the nearby Bandemere Speedway. Green Mountain Trail intersects again with Hayden Trail; stay right on Green Mountain Trail. Continue down the trail, reach a T, and turn left, staying on Green Mountain Trail. At 2.86 miles, the trail empties into a small gully. There is a small, cruel spurt of uphill and then the trail heads back down to the trailhead, coming out on the opposite side of the parking lot from where you started.

NEARBY ATTRACTIONS

North Dinosaur Open Space Park, Rooney Hogback Open Space Park, and Loveland Trail Open Space Park; for more information, visit the Web site for the city of Lakewood: **lakewood.org**.

Matthews/Winters Open Space Park; for more information, visit the Web site for Jefferson County Open Space: **jeffco.us/openspace**.

MEYER RANCH OPEN SPACE PARK: LODGEPOLE LOOP

23

IN BRIEF

Meyer Ranch is a wonderful family, novice hiking area with easy trails and plentiful picnic sites. The Lodgepole Loop is true to its nomenclature, as the pines dominate the route. Add-on trails render this an ideal spot for hardy and adventurous hikers. The all-year access plus moderate crowds make this a well-rounded area desirable to all.

DESCRIPTION

Depart the parking lot and travel a short way to the trailhead kiosk. Walk through the meadow, toward the bathroom, located far from the trailhead. Leave the service road–like trail, turn right, and head to the left side of Owl's Perch Trail. Pass the first of many picnic-table sites on the right and travel along a well-maintained, singletrack hiking path. Owl's Perch Trail loops around the picnic area, but both the left and right access lead to Lodgepole Loop.

At the intersection of Owl's Perch Trail and Lodgepole Loop, take a right. Travel along until the trail forks at a service road and a hiking path. Take a right onto the hiking path and follow the arrows that mark the trail, which drops right into a meadow and passes a bench. The path travels through a few switchbacks as

KEY AT-A-GLANCE INFORMATION

LENGTH: 2 miles
CONFIGURATION: Balloon
DIFFICULTY: Easy
SCENERY: Heavily forested with lodgepole pine trees
EXPOSURE: Shaded
TRAFFIC: Moderate
TRAIL SURFACE: Smooth and hard-packed dirt
HIKING TIME: 1 hour
SEASON: All year
ACCESS: Free; open sunrise to sunset
MAPS: USGS Conifer
FACILITIES: Restrooms, picnic facilities
SPECIAL COMMENTS: Dogs are allowed but must be leashed. No hunting or overnight camping. The Meyer family still owns and resides in the historic Victorian home adjacent to the park on the north side of US 285. Please respect their privacy.

Directions

From Denver, take C 470 south for 6 miles to US 285. Follow US 285 west for 11.5 miles until it intersects with South Turkey Creek Road. Turn right at signs for Meyer Ranch Open Space, and follow the road under the highway to the parking lot.

GPS Trailhead Coordinates

UTM Zone (WGS84)   13S
Easting   0476650
Northing   4377180
Latitude   N 39.543974°
Longitude   W 105.271749°

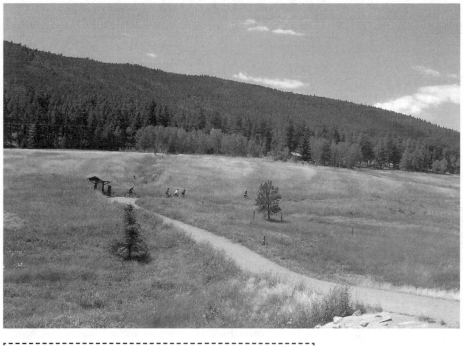

Mountain bikers leave the trailhead at Meyer Ranch Open Space.

it goes into thick forest. Pass the spur for Sunny Aspen Trail on the right. This trail eventually meets up with Old Ski Run Trail. A portion of what is now Meyer Ranch was used in the early 1940s as a ski hill. Remnants are still visible in the upper end of the park, now a forested aspen grove.

The Lodgepole Loop continues through dense forest, with cool patches of shade, and crosses through a small, open meadow area. If you encounter a circus animal, do not be alarmed. Legend has it that the ranch served as winter quarters for animals of the P.T. Barnum Circus in the late 1880s. (When the Meyers remodeled the ranch house in 1995, they found a board with the inscription "Circus Town, 1889.")

Pass a second spur for Sunny Aspen Trail on the right. Continue straight on Lodgepole Loop and dip down, crossing shaded stairs over a small, wet gully. The trail is a roller coaster, going up and down, but never at a large descent or ascent. A few gentle switchbacks through the lodgepoles lead down to familiar territory. Back at the Owl's Perch Trail, take a right (or left) and head back to the restrooms, trailhead, and parking lot.

NEARBY ATTRACTIONS

Other Jefferson County Open Space hikes: **jeffco.us/openspace**.

24 MOUNT EVANS WILDERNESS: HELL'S HOLE TRAIL

KEY AT-A-GLANCE INFORMATION

LENGTH: 9.32 miles

CONFIGURATION: Out-and-back

DIFFICULTY: Difficult

SCENERY: Dense forest that opens to views of high mountain peaks

EXPOSURE: Mostly shaded

TRAFFIC: Moderate

TRAIL SURFACE: Hard-packed dirt, rocky

HIKING TIME: 4.5 hours

SEASON: June–October

ACCESS: Free

MAPS: USGS Georgetown

FACILITIES: Restrooms, picnic areas

SPECIAL COMMENTS: Although access is free, users must obtain a wilderness usage permit at the trailhead. Dogs are allowed but must be leashed. Bicycles and any motorized vehicle are not permitted.

IN BRIEF

Don't let the name of this hike deter. Hell's Hole is a difficult hike, but its challenge is rewarded. This trail travels through the woods to a high alpine basin in the Mount Evans Wilderness. When it ends at Hell's Hole, the path opens to a meadow where alpine willows grow in the shadow of Gray Wolf Mountain and Mount Evans. The only hell of the day will be found in the busy passing lanes of I-70 on the way there.

DESCRIPTION

Hell's Hole Trail #53 starts by traveling through the Chicago Creek picnic area, surrounded by pine trees. The trail is not well defined at first, so walk uphill, stay to the left going toward the creek, and then enter an aspen grove. Here, the trail is easier to find and travels along West Chicago Creek for about a mile.

Around five minutes into the hike, a self-issuing permit station seems to come out of nowhere. Registration is mandatory. No fees or quotas exist, but the Forest Service tracks how many people use this trail and what they do here, so just fill out the form, deposit the white slip below, and keep the tag.

Follow the trail through several large groves of aspen trees, and cross the small creek

GPS Trailhead Coordinates

UTM Zone (WGS84) 13S

Easting   0443648

Northing 4392349

Latitude N 39.679111°

Longitude W 105.657103°

Directions

From Denver, take I-70 west to Idaho Springs (exit 240). Go left, traveling south on CO 103, which is also Mount Evans Road. Go 6.5 miles, and take a right at the sign for Chicago Creek Campground. Go 3 miles on West Chicago Creek Road. The trailhead is at the end of the road.

N

0   0.4   0.8
mile

Independence
Mtn.

To
Idaho Springs

P

Lake
Edith

Little Sugarloaf
Peak

Sugarloaf
Peak

West Chicago Creek

MOUNT EVANS
WILDERNESS

Hell's
Hole

Gray Wolf
Mtn.

The gnarled trunk of a bristlecone pine at timberline and the turnaround for Hell's Hole.

two times. These aspen trees are bent way over to the left and look like a big gust of wind once came through here and tried to blow them all down.

The trail alternates between steep, rocky sections and smooth, level sections for most of the hike. After a half hour, you officially enter Mount Evans Wilderness. Views open up a little toward the left as the trees begin to transition from aspens to evergreens, which thin with elevation. There are views in all directions. The tall mountain that you have been able to see for most of this hike is Mount Evans. The last mile of the trail is a gentle grade at tree line that ends at a valley with small ponds and oddly shaped, big trees with bushy tops called bristlecone pines. Mount Evans is still off to the left and the dominant mountain. Gray Wolf Mountain sits to the right and is closer to this trail. Once you arrive at the base of Gray Wolf Mountain, the trail ends at the meadow area called Hell's Hole. From here, turn around and head back the way you came.

NEARBY ATTRACTIONS

Mount Evans Wilderness hikes: **fs.fed.us/r2/arnf** (reference Clear Creek Ranger District) or **tinyurl.com/ye2m26m**.

MOUNT EVANS WILDERNESS: MOUNT BIERSTADT

25

IN BRIEF

Mount Bierstadt and Mount Evans are two of the closest fourteeners to Denver. (A fourteener is any mountain peak above 14,000 feet.) Mount Bierstadt is easy to find and fairly easy to navigate. The trail is steep in places. A 3-mile summit reached from the Guanella Pass approach is a great way to start an addiction to the Colorado fourteeners.

DESCRIPTION

Set out on Mount Bierstadt Trail #711 and deposit the required wilderness usage permit in the drop box. The hike starts above tree line and takes you through the largest willow bog in Colorado. A boardwalk has been built to protect the alpine willows and to keep hikers' feet dry from the bog that dominates the first 1.5 miles of the hike. The boardwalk has made rather difficult terrain manageable; otherwise, the trail is well defined, with stable, packed dirt and some rocks.

The first 1.5 miles are also a steady descent from the trailhead, passing Deadmans Lake on the left and continuing to the Scott Gomer Creek crossing.

KEY AT-A-GLANCE INFORMATION

LENGTH: 6 miles, or 7.4 miles with Sawtooth Ridge option
CONFIGURATION: Out-and-back
DIFFICULTY: Difficult
SCENERY: Alpine tundra, high mountain peaks
EXPOSURE: Heavily exposed due to high altitude
TRAFFIC: Heavy
TRAIL SURFACE: Hard-packed dirt, extremely rocky, large talus
HIKING TIME: 4 hours
SEASON: June–October
ACCESS: Free; open sunrise to sunset
MAPS: USGS Evans and Georgetown
FACILITIES: None
SPECIAL COMMENTS: Although access is free, users must obtain a wilderness usage permit at the trailhead. Dogs must be leashed. Bicycles and any motorized vehicles are not permitted.

Directions

From Denver, take I-70 west to Georgetown (exit 228). Go down the exit ramp, turn left under I-70, then turn right at Argentine Street and follow the signs leading to Guanella Pass. Stay left at a fork in the road, and at Rose Street turn right. Go through the next stop sign; the road turns to the left and becomes Guanella Pass Road. Take this road 10 miles to Mount Evans Wilderness. The road becomes dirt but is passable by most passenger cars. The trailhead is on the east side of the road.

GPS Trailhead Coordinates

UTM Zone (WGS84)   13S
Easting   0439060
Northing   4382960
Latitude   N 39.594204°
Longitude   W 105.709733°

N

| 0 | 0.4 | 0.8 |

mile

Summit Lake

Mount Evans

West Ridge Trl.

Mount Spalding

Abyss Lake

West Ridge Trl.

Sawtooth Ridge Trl.

Mount Bierstadt

Frozen Lake

Mount Bierstadt Trl.

MOUNT EVANS WILDERNESS

Scott Gomer Creek

Deadmans Lake

P

To Georgetown

Guanella Pass

FEET

14,000

13,500

13,000

12,500

12,000

11,500

11,000

10,500

10,000

0.5   1   1.5   2   2.5   3

MILES

Two more fourteeners, Grays Peak and Torreys Peak, can be seen in the distance from Mount Bierstadt.

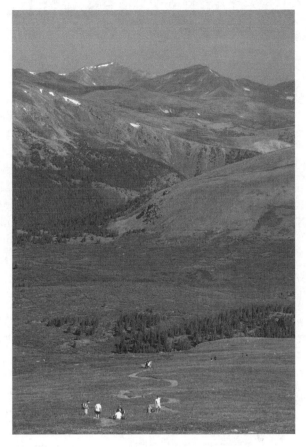

At the fork in the trail, veer right on the more heavily used trail. Here is a good place to stop and appreciate the view of Mount Bierstadt and the Sawtooth Ridge. Once the willows fade away, the trail becomes steep and continues in a southeastern direction. As the trail winds up the west-facing slope of Mount Bierstadt, keep an eye out for marmots or pikas. At 13,760 feet, turn northeast and hike along the ridge. Most landmarks along this entire trail are marked by cairns.

The summit is only 0.25 miles away right after where the willow trees fade away from the trail. The terrain is characterized by larger talus, and hikers must scramble over a few. At the 14,060-foot summit of Mount Bierstadt, relish the panoramic view. To the northwest, two more fourteeners are visible: Grays Peak (14,270 feet) and Torreys Peak (14,267 feet). To the east, you can see Abyss Lake.

From the summit you can take the Sawtooth Ridge option (see page 108), which connects hikers to the summit of Mount Evans. Or turn around from here and head back 3 miles to the trailhead.

NEARBY ATTRACTIONS

Mount Evans Wilderness hikes: **fs.fed.us/r2/arnf** (reference Clear Creek Ranger District).

26 MOUNT EVANS WILDERNESS: MOUNT EVANS

KEY AT-A-GLANCE INFORMATION

LENGTH: Sawtooth option: 1.5 miles one way (add on to Bierstadt summit); West Ridge option: 9 miles

CONFIGURATION: Sawtooth: balloon; West Ridge: out-and-back

DIFFICULTY: Difficult

SCENERY: Alpine tundra and high mountain peaks

EXPOSURE: Heavily exposed due to high altitude

TRAFFIC: Heavy

TRAIL SURFACE: Hard-packed dirt, extremely rocky, large talus

HIKING TIME: 4.5 hours

SEASON: June–October

ACCESS: Free; open sunrise to sunset

MAPS: USGS Evans and Georgetown

FACILITIES: None

SPECIAL COMMENTS: Sawtooth option: Mount Bierstadt summit to Mount Evans summit via Sawtooth Ridge is 1.5 miles one way, plus the 3 miles one way to Mount Bierstadt's summit. West Ridge option: Uses the Guanella Pass trailhead, same trailhead as Mount Bierstadt, but reaches the summit via a different, 9-mile route. Although access is free, users must obtain a wilderness usage permit at the trailhead. Dogs must be leashed. No bikes or motorized vehicles.

IN BRIEF

There are approximately 12 different ways to reach this fourteener summit. The Sawtooth option allows hikers to summit two fourteeners in one day—both Mount Bierstadt and Mount Evans. Generally, summit Mount Bierstadt first and then Mount Evans since the peaks are 1.5 miles apart. The West Ridge option is a good out-and-back hike on the less popular side of Mount Evans. Most tourists access Mount Evans from Echo Lake or Mount Evans Road on the east and northeast side.

DESCRIPTION

SAWTOOTH OPTION:

Hike to the summit of Mount Bierstadt (see page 105) and head north toward the Sawtooth Ridge. The trail along the Sawtooth is not as harrowing as it may appear. Lightning storms are more frequent after noon, so assess the weather, the time, and your physical condition at this point.

Begin descending to the north on the east side of the Sawtooth Ridge. Pass through talus and be prepared to do some light scrambling. Follow the cairns as they direct hikers to a point below a significant saddle. From here,

---

GPS Trailhead Coordinates

UTM Zone (WGS84) 13S

Easting   0439060

Northing 4382960

Latitude N 39.594204°

Longitude W 105.709733°

Directions ⟶

From Denver, take I-70 west to Georgetown (exit 228). Go down the exit ramp, turn left under I-70, then turn right at Argentine Street and follow the signs leading to Guanella Pass. Stay left at a fork in the road, and at Rose Street turn right. Go through the next stop sign; the road turns to the left and becomes Guanella Pass Road. Take this road 10 miles to Mount Evans Wilderness. The road becomes dirt but is passable by most passenger cars. The trailhead is on the east side of the road.

N

0   0.4   0.8
mile

Summit
Lake

Mount
Evans

West Ridge Trl.

Mount
Spalding

Abyss
Lake

West Ridge Trl.

Sawtooth Ridge Trl.

Mount
Bierstadt

Frozen
Lake

Mount Bierstadt Trl.

MOUNT EVANS
WILDERNESS

Sawtooth Option

Scott Gomer Creek

Deadmans
Lake

Guanella
Pass

To
Georgetown

14,500

14,000

13,500

13,000

12,500

FEET

12,000

11,500

11,000

10,500

MT. BIERSTADT

MT. EVANS

RETURN VIA
WEST RIDGE

2   4   6   8   10   11.5

MILES

regain elevation as you approach the saddle. Cross over the saddle to the west side of the Sawtooth Ridge. Continue to follow the cairns along a wide ledge and across a gully of smaller, loose rock. You will now encounter a ledge that ascends diagonally across a cliff band. The ledge is exposed, so take your time and mind your footing.

Just beyond the Sawtooth is a gentle slope comprised of tundra and sporadic boulders. Follow this slope to the east as you prepare for the last segment of scrambling up the west ridge of Mount Evans. At 14,264 feet, you have accomplished a difficult task. Two fourteeners in one day! Be prepared to see people who have walked the few hundred feet up from the parking lot. Yes, there is a parking lot, observatory, and paved road that lead all the way up to Mount Evans on this side. Retrace your steps or hike down Mount Evans as detailed in the West Ridge option below.

WEST RIDGE OPTION:

Set out on Mount Bierstadt Trail #711 and deposit the required wilderness usage permit in the drop box. The hike starts above tree line and takes you through the largest willow bog in Colorado. A boardwalk has been built to protect the alpine willows and to keep hikers' feet dry from the bog that dominates the first 1.5 miles of the hike. The boardwalk has made rather difficult terrain manageable; otherwise, the trail is well defined, with stable, packed dirt and some rocks.

The first 1.5 miles are also a steady descent from the trailhead, passing Deadmans Lake on the left and continuing to the Scott Gomer Creek crossing.

At the fork in the trail, go left. (Mount Bierstadt hikers go right.)

Pass the cliff walls that extend 1 mile north of Sawtooth and come to the open tundra of Mount Spalding. Cross to the south side of Spalding's ridge, pass Spalding's summit, and reach the west end of Mount Evans at 13,900 feet. Scramble approximately 1 mile to Mount Evans's summit. Most of this traverse is on solid talus rock. After reaching the summit, turn around and head back the way you came to the trailhead.

NEARBY ATTRACTIONS

Mount Evans Wilderness hikes: **fs.fed.us/r2/arnf** (reference Clear Creek Ranger District).

MOUNT FALCON PARK: CASTLE AND PARMALEE TRAIL LOOP

27

IN BRIEF

Mount Falcon Open Space Park is an easily accessible hike from Denver that includes a blood-pumping climb through open meadows, ponderosa pine trees, and seasonal wildflowers. This trail covers most of the 11.1 miles of trails in Mount Falcon. Castle Trail leads from the plains to the foothills on a narrow road that once carried Stanley Steamer automobiles.

DESCRIPTION

From the trailhead, take the well-marked Castle Trail. The view is dominated by Red Rocks Open Space and the Red Rocks amphitheater across the valley. Glance back for a view of downtown Denver. Quickly come to the intersection where Turkey Trot Trail, a hiker-only path, goes off to the right. Stay on Castle Trail, bearing left. Wind up the hillside going through yuccas, oak trees, sage, and non-native thistles, considered an invasive species and quite a nuisance here. At many points, the ascent levels out, and it feels as though you've reached the top of the hill. Pass the point in the trail where the Turkey Trot Trail reemerges and still you have quite a ways to go up the hill.

The cars in the trailhead parking lot become mere specks. On a clear day, the views

KEY AT-A-GLANCE INFORMATION

LENGTH: 9.5 miles

CONFIGURATION: Balloon

DIFFICULTY: Difficult

SCENERY: Scenic vistas, plains, foothills; mix of meadows and forests

EXPOSURE: Mostly exposed, shade in higher sections

TRAFFIC: Heavy

TRAIL SURFACE: Dirt, loose rocks

HIKING TIME: 5 hours

SEASON: All year

ACCESS: Free; open sunrise to sunset

MAPS: USGS Morrison and Indian Hills

FACILITIES: Restrooms, picnic shelter, information kiosk

SPECIAL COMMENTS: Dogs must be leashed. Traffic is heavy on this trail, especially with mountain bikes and athletes. It is not uncommon to see a person ride the trail, put the bike back in the car, and then turn around and run the same trail.

Directions

From Denver, take I-70 west to the Morrison/Golden exit and CO 26. Take a left, traveling west on CO 26 for 4 miles to the town of Morrison. Go right into downtown Morrison on Main Street. Go left at CO 8 at the end of Morrison town and travel 1.6 miles to Forest Avenue. Turn right on Forest Avenue and follow the signs for Mount Falcon Open Space.

GPS Trailhead Coordinates

UTM Zone (WGS84) 13S

Easting 0483070

Northing 4388340

Latitude N 39.644680°

Longitude W 105.197318°

expand many miles to the east over the Colorado prairie. The white dots, farther past downtown Denver, are the white tentlike spires of Denver International Airport. Climbing higher and higher, you are rewarded by seasonal wildflowers, including columbines and Indian paintbrushes.

A picnic shelter marks the true top of the hill and the intersection with the Walker's Dream Trail. Continue straight on the main Castle Trail and pass the Two-Dog Trail on the left.

From this point forward, the trail is wider, smoother, and easier to navigate. The trees also offer more shade. Travel another 0.5 miles and continue straight past the intersection with Meadow Trail. After another 0.4 miles, take a right where the Meadow Trail merges with the Castle Trail. You are on a smooth, well-maintained service road. On the left are remnants of a 1989 forest fire along with signs of new vegetation in the form of wildflowers.

Arrive at the opposite trailhead for Mount Falcon Park on the western side of the park. Near the restroom, take a left onto Parmalee Trail and travel on this trail for 2 miles.

The trail immediately descends through lush forest and gives you a nice break from sun on a hot day. The trail levels and gradually ascends across an open hillside. Turn right onto Meadow Trail, passing Mount Falcon on the left. Merge again in 0.3 miles with the Castle Trail and end the small balloon portion of the hike. Take a right and proceed down the long hill, back the way you came, all the way to the parking lot.

NEARBY ATTRACTIONS

Other Jefferson County area hikes, including nearby Lair O' the Bear Park and Matthews/Winters Open Space Park: **jeffco.us/openspace**.

28 RED ROCKS: TRADING POST TRAIL

KEY AT-A-GLANCE INFORMATION

LENGTH: 1.46 miles

CONFIGURATION: Loop

DIFFICULTY: Easy

SCENERY: Smooth, red stones; large rock walls; small trees and brush

EXPOSURE: Virtually no shade

TRAFFIC: Heavy

TRAIL SURFACE: Dirt

HIKING TIME: 1.5 hours

SEASON: All year

ACCESS: Free; open 5 a.m. to 30 minutes after sunset

MAPS: USGS Morrison

FACILITIES: Store, restrooms, restaurant, amphitheater, picnic shelter

SPECIAL COMMENTS: In the event of a live performance, visitors to the park will be instructed as to when the park will close. Most concerts are in the evenings. Dogs are allowed but must be on a six-foot leash. Do not climb or rappel off the red rocks; you'll face a $999 fine or 180 days in jail. No horses or bikes are allowed.

IN BRIEF

Red Rocks Park is a well-known venue for Colorado's best outdoor concerts. The natural rock that jettisons out of the hillside is flaming red and attracts music lovers in the summer and outdoor enthusiasts all year. The Trading Post Trail offers an opportunity to pass through spectacular rock formations and catch a peek at the amphitheater.

DESCRIPTION

The trail starts at the Trading Post Store traveling along the road on the northern side of the store; the trail leaves this roadside quickly. Take the northernmost entrance to the Trading Post Trail, which is on the right side of the Trading Post. The Red Rocks Pueblo, now commonly known as the Trading Post, is a registered Denver landmark. You immediately pass the rocks that line the southern side of the amphitheater. The trail runs along Ship Rock Road and past the upper south parking lot.

Enter low-lying brush as the trail begins a slight descent. It is extremely crowded on weekends and mostly crowded any other time. The red-dirt path is wide enough for one person. Expect to kick up plenty of red dust if conditions are dry.

GPS Trailhead Coordinates

UTM Zone (WGS84) 13S

Easting   0482660

Northing 4390260

Latitude N 39.661972°

Longitude W 105.202147°

Directions

From Denver, take I-70 west to the Morrison exit and CO 26. Go left, traveling south on CO 26 to Red Rocks Park. Take the first park entrance on the right, West Alameda Parkway. Turn left on Trading Post Road, and park at the Trading Post Store.

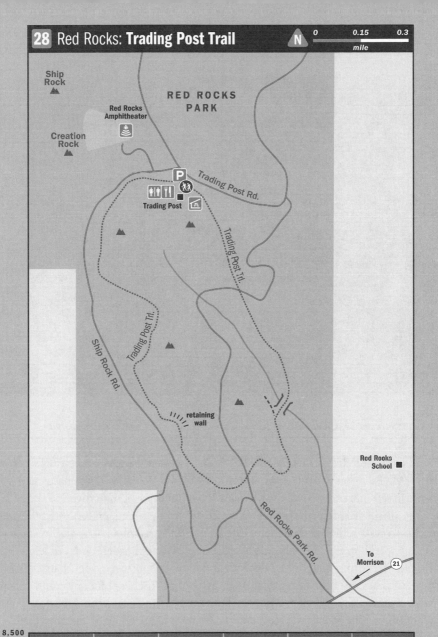

N

0   0.15   0.3
mile

Ship
Rock

RED ROCKS
PARK

Red Rocks
Amphitheater

Creation
Rock

P

Trading Post Rd.

Trading Post

Trading Post Trl.

Trading Post Trl.

Ship Rock Rd.

retaining
wall

Red Rocks
School

Red Rocks Park Rd.

To
Morrison   21

FEET

8,500
8,000
7,500
7,000
6,500
6,000
5,500
5,000
4,500

0.25   0.5   0.75   1   1.25   1.46
MILES

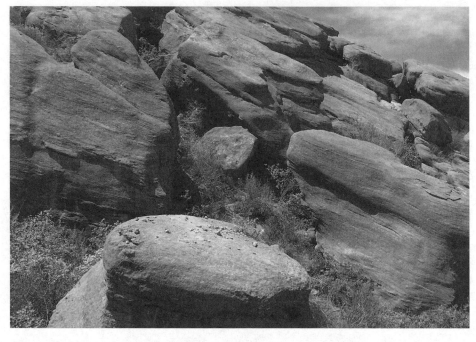

One of the many large, red rock boulder fields along Trading Post Trail in Red Rocks Park.

To the left are moderate-sized versions of the red rocks rocketing out toward the trail. Pass these formations and descend several sets of man-made stairs. The trail is well marked with signs that say "trail" and have an arrow.

Cross a wooden bridge with a small stream that runs underneath, flanked by rocks. Cross another man-made bridge over a dry streambed. The trail widens for a moment, and hikers can walk side by side. You're again bordered on the left by large, red boulder formations. In the distance is a view of southwest suburban Denver.

You may spot an occasional deer, as well as finches, blue jays, and magpies. Most noteworthy are sightings of mountain bluebirds and the American kestrel. Wild plum, chokecherry trees, and evening primrose grow in this prairie-to-mountain transition zone. The trees you see include mahogany, sumac, cottonwood, and ponderosa pine.

The trail turns into disintegrated asphalt that was once the main road. Stay on the asphalt portion of trail; do not veer to the left, where trail erosion has occurred. You will still be walking along smooth curvatures of the red rock formations. The trail continues to descend at a more gradual pace, where stairs are not needed. An open meadow appears on the left, and drought-resistant plants such as yucca mark the trail. Keep in mind that running a counterclockwise version of this trail means that hikers have fewer uphill climbs and more downhill walks.

Pass a man-made retaining wall on the left. This a good place to stop and look at the views. The trail turns to the left and starts another descent, heading

Red Rocks is famous for its rock formations. Remember to just look up and don't touch.

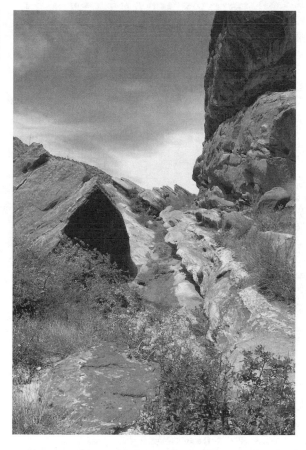

directly to a long, red wall of rock. Keep winding down, down, down.

Cross another man-made bridge with a creek running underneath. At the bottom of the hill, cross Red Rocks Park Road and watch for traffic. The trail widens, and loose, red dirt borders miniature wildflowers, grass, and shrubbery.

On the left, pass a sign marked DANGER RATTLE-SNAKE AREA—CLOSED. To the right you'll see an area that has been fenced off for restoration. Farther to the right is an elementary school. At a fork in the road, take a right toward the bridge and pass an old incinerator on the left. Cross a man-made bridge that is high over a creek. The trail begins to ascend gradually. As it does, a hillside of brush and yucca appears on the right. To the left is a little drop-off. Take the man-made stairs and cross Red Rocks Park Road again. After crossing the road, climb another set of man-made stairs. The trail continues to travel alongside a drastic drop-off, and posted DANGER DROP-OFF signs mean what they say. Scramble across a long section of flat, red rock. Continue to the right and stay on the trail, even when you see a turnoff to the left. The Trading Post will be straight ahead. Take a right to get off the trail, and you're free to explore some more.

NEARBY ATTRACTIONS

Dakota Ridge Trail, Red Rocks Trail: **denvergov.org; redrocksonline.com; dinoridge.org.** Matthews/Winters Open Space Park, Dinosaur Ridge: **jeffco.us/ openspace.**

29 ROCKY MOUNTAIN ARSENAL NATIONAL WILDLIFE REFUGE: LAKES LOOP

KEY AT-A-GLANCE INFORMATION

LENGTH: 1.7 miles

CONFIGURATION: Loop

DIFFICULTY: Easy

SCENERY: Barren prairie, some grasses; lakes and cottonwood trees

EXPOSURE: Full exposure; some shade in cottonwood trees

TRAFFIC: Moderate

TRAIL SURFACE: Smooth, hard-packed dirt; asphalt

HIKING TIME: 1 hour

SEASON: All year; some closures April 15–Oct. 15

ACCESS: Free; trails open Tuesday, Wednesday, Saturday, and Sunday, excluding holidays, 6 a.m.–6 p.m.

MAPS: USGS Montbello

FACILITIES: Restrooms, picnic facilities; visitor center with interpretive nature displays and activities

SPECIAL COMMENTS: Dogs, horses, and bikes not allowed. Assistance dogs welcome. It is illegal to keep eagle feathers found here. Call the visitor center at (303) 289-0930 to make a reservation for the two-hour trolley wildlife viewing tour at 10 a.m. on Wednesdays, Saturdays, and Sundays. Special emergency response procedures are detailed on the map at the visitor center.

IN BRIEF

This barren and deserted former Army arsenal and chemical munitions facility gives some visitors an eerie feeling. Weapons were produced here during WWII, and then the land was leased to commercial pesticide companies. It is the largest contiguous open space in the Denver metropolitan area, and the site is undergoing a major environmental restoration. No sign of such activity can be seen on this short and sweet hike around two beautiful lakes, even over one of the lakes. But the whisper of ghosts may quicken your stride.

DESCRIPTION

Leave the visitor center and travel south 0.1 mile until the trail merges with Prairie Trail. Take an immediate left, then continue until the trail splits around Lake Mary. Lined by railroad ties, the dirt trail is dusty in dry summer. At the Lake Mary fork, turn right onto Lake Mary Trail and travel counterclockwise around the lake.

The trail is heavily exposed at first, but near the lake, you enter a nice respite in a cluster of cottonwoods. Continue the trip around Lake Mary and ignore the spurs and trail intersections that take hikers away from the lake.

On the southwest side of Lake Mary, take a right onto Prairie Trail. Here, the trail is again

GPS Trailhead Coordinates

UTM Zone (WGS84) 13S

Easting   0511800

Northing   4407660

Latitude   N 39.818843°

Longitude   W 104.862125°

Directions

From Denver, take I-70 east to the Havana Street exit. Go left, traveling north, cross over 56th Avenue, and enter the refuge. All visitors enter by passing a deserted military-guard station. Pass through and continue to the visitor center for mandatory check-in.

N

0   0.1   0.2
mile

ROCKY MOUNTAIN
ARSENAL NATIONAL
WILDLIFE REFUGE

Sand Creek Lateral Ditch

Visitor
Center

P

Lake Mary

Lake Ladora

Havana St.

Lake Ladora Trl.

Prairie Trl.

Shuttle
Stop

P

E. 64th Ave.

To
Denver

FEET

8,500
8,000
7,500
7,000
6,500
6,000
5,500
5,000
4,500

0.25   0.5   0.75   1   1.25   1.5   1.7
MILES

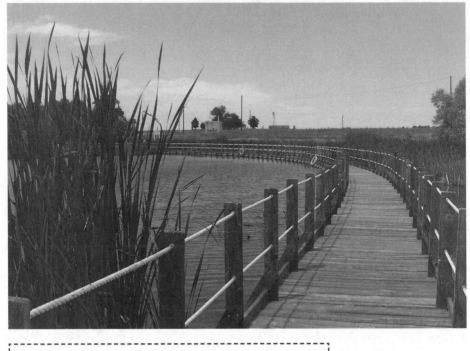

Lakes Loop offers hikers a chance to cross Lake Mary on a boardwalk.

exposed, dry prairie land. You quickly come to a switchback built into a berm. After climbing up and over it, travel along a ridge, and walk through high prairie grasses.

At the intersection of Prairie Trail and Sixth Avenue, take a left turn onto Sixth Avenue. Follow it for a short distance, and then turn left into the shuttle-stop parking area, where there is a restroom and trailhead kiosk.

Go around the kiosk and enter the Lake Ladora Trail. This trail has nesting closures from October 15 to April 15, so check at the visitor center or call ahead. Pass a fork in the trail as the path approaches Lake Ladora. Take a left turn here and travel clockwise around Lake Ladora. Pass beneath lakeside native cotton-woods, used by cavity nesting flickers and prey-seeking hawks.

Lake Ladora, a man-made reservoir, provides habitat for many wildlife species that could not have lived here when it was an arsenal. Again, the trail departs from the lake and merges with a service road, where you turn right. Cross the road diagonally, and take a left onto the trail that leads hikers back to Lake Mary. The trail splits again, almost immediately, to take you on Lake Mary Trail either direction. Take a left, pass a bull-frog sign, and take an almost immediate right on the portion of the trail that crosses directly over Lake Mary. Stroll along the floating boardwalk as it moves with every step. After crossing the bridge spanning Lake Mary, take a right at a familiar intersection and follow the trail to the left to the visitor center.

NEARBY ATTRACTIONS

Other Rocky Mountain Arsenal hikes: **fws.gov/rockymountainarsenal.**

WESTMINSTER: COLORADO HILLS TRAIL 30

IN BRIEF

Those who like quiet solitude will enjoy the lake at Mower Reservoir. Walk 1.5 miles one way through Westminster's Colorado Hills Open Space to reach this beautiful 11-acre pond. In the early summer, wildflowers bloom from the trailhead to the lake. Most people come here to give the dogs some exercise and barely venture past the irrigation ditch. Dogs must be leashed outside of the dog park.

DESCRIPTION

Leave the parking area and go through the fence to the right of the trail kiosk. Note any posted rattlesnake warnings since this trail is rumored to be full of them. The first portion is a 20-acre off-leash, fenced dog park. The wide trail is mostly dirt and small, loose rocks.

Walk westward toward the power line and mountain views. Ahead is a bench and a small shelter; pass them on the right. Come to an irrigation ditch and a small pond, and take a left across the bridge that spans the canal. After the bridge, take a right and continue to head through the grassy hills at a slight incline as the trail narrows. On the right, the canal and pond are still visible. To the left are power lines and an arid yucca field. In the mornings, songbirds call out across the meadow.

KEY AT-A-GLANCE INFORMATION

LENGTH: 4.4 miles

CONFIGURATION: Reverse balloon

DIFFICULTY: Easy

SCENERY: Pond ringed with cottonwood trees, tall grasses, irrigation ditch, views of mountains

EXPOSURE: No shade

TRAFFIC: Heavy in dog park, mild otherwise

TRAIL SURFACE: Dirt

HIKING TIME: 1.5 hours

SEASON: All year

ACCESS: Free; sunrise to sunset

MAPS: USGS Louisville

FACILITIES: Kiosk

SPECIAL COMMENTS: No facilities at this trailhead. The first portion of the hike is a 20-acre, off-leash dog park. It is very crowded before 9 a.m. and after 5 p.m. on weekdays and all day on weekends.

For information on hiking trails at Standley Lake and other Westminster lakes and open space, visit the city of Westminster's Web site: ci.westminster.co.us.

The Rocky Flats National Wildlife Refuge is managed by the US Fish and Wildlife Service: fws.gov/rockyflats.

Directions

From Denver, take I-25 north to CO 36, exit at Church Ranch Road, and go left. When you cross CO 121, Church Ranch Road turns into West 100th Avenue. The road curves sharply to the right onto Simms Street. Look for 106th Avenue on the right, and turn into the trailhead parking lot on the left.

GPS Trailhead Coordinates

UTM Zone (WGS84) 13S

Easting   0488897

Northing   4415222

Latitude   N 39.886986°

Longitude   W 105.129859°

N

0   0.15   0.3

mile

Simms St.

P

Off-leash
dog park

W. 107th Ave.

canal

To Church
Ranch Rd.
and Westminster

W. 100th Ave.

W. 96th Ave.

Mower
Reservoir

8,500
8,000
7,500
7,000
6,500
6,000
5,500
5,000
4,500

FEET

1   2   3   4   4.4

MILES

Mower Reservoir is but a pond, but a lovely little body of water. In addition to being a nice respite, this is your turnaround point on Colorado Hills Trail.

The dirt path meanders, then widens into a dirt road. Curve a little to the left and begin to see unobstructed views of the Boulder Flatirons and all of its neighboring mountain peaks.

Plane traffic may rumble overhead from the small planes that fly in and out of Jefferson County Airport, which is directly behind your right shoulder. Look over your left shoulder at views of Standley Lake, Denver metro area's second-largest lake after Barr Lake.

Come to a trail crossing and take a right at the sign that points to Mower Reservoir. The trail descends a little at this point. Prairie-dog mounds line the trail, and constant prairie-dog chatter fills the air. Beyond Colorado Hills, to the west of Mower Reservoir, is the Rocky Flats National Wildlife Refuge, which you can see from here. This 6,250-acre wildlife refuge replaced the controversial nuclear disposal plant and its buffer land.

Go through a gate, pass a barbed-wire fence, and continue. Mower Reservoir comes into view on the left. Reach the crest of the hill and descend toward the pond. Catch-and-release fishing is allowed, but bait fishing is prohibited at the lake. Take a respite and watch waterfowl or sit in the shade of the cottonwood trees.

Trace back to where you came from and go back through the gate. At the top of the hill, go right to make a loop back to the trailhead. A Mower Reservoir directional sign is posted here, where we originally turned right to get to the lake.

The trail makes a wide arc around to the right and circles back to the left. The landscape is still grass and shrubby meadow, and larger views of Standley Lake are to the right. Houses come into view as the trail goes to the left. Crest a hill and spot the dog park on the right. Take the trail down the hillside as it reconnects at the canal and pond. Go right and back to the trailhead. Deposit any extra water into the dishes provided for furry companions at the trailhead.

31 WHITE RANCH PARK: BELCHER HILL

KEY AT-A-GLANCE INFORMATION

LENGTH: 4.84 miles

CONFIGURATION: Out-and-back, loop

DIFFICULTY: Difficult

SCENERY: Meadow; views of Denver, Golden, Ralston Reservoir; passes through forest and grassy plains

EXPOSURE: Sunny in meadow portion; cool, shaded in forested areas

TRAFFIC: Heavy; popular with mountain bikers

TRAIL SURFACE: Rocky, hard-packed, and very steep

HIKING TIME: 3.5 hours

SEASON: All year

ACCESS: Free; open 1 hour before sunrise to 1 hour after sunset

MAPS: Park map at trailhead

FACILITIES: Restroom, picnic table, barbecue grill

SPECIAL COMMENTS: Take plenty of breaks and drink plenty of water on this unforgiving climb. Dogs must be leashed, fires prohibited, no vehicles, hiking by permit only, bikes yield to all, no hunting, no firearms, no feeding wildlife, and no collection of natural resources (wildflowers). A complete list of regulations is at the trailhead kiosk.

IN BRIEF

Belcher Hill is a small part of the 19.7 miles of trails that comprise White Ranch Park. This long, rocky, and very steep trail has great views.

DESCRIPTION

Pass the trailhead kiosk to the White Ranch Park Jefferson County Open Space sign and gate. Go through the gate and close it behind you. Here the trail is arid and narrow, with room for only one hiker to pass at a time. Rocks and dirt are evenly spaced, yet the ground is hard-packed.

White Ranch Park was first settled in 1865 by immigrants James and Mary Bond after their son was killed under their wagon wheel en route to California. In 1913, Paul and Anna Lee White purchased part of the land and operated a cattle ranch until 1969. Anna Lee White gave the land to Jefferson County Open Space and dedicated White Ranch Park to the memory of Paul White in 1975.

You face an elevation gain of 1,800 feet on this trail; don't let its beginning fool you. Mountain-biking bloggers comment that this trail is "one of the best for quad and lung burners" or "long, busting climbs that will make you want to puke!"

GPS Trailhead Coordinates

UTM Zone (WGS84)   13S

Easting   0478760

Northing   4405240

Latitude   N 39.796856°

Longitude   W 105.248096°

Directions

From Denver, take I-70 west and travel 3.5 miles to CO 58. Exit CO 58, going west toward Golden/Central City. Travel 5.4 miles on CO 58, then turn right onto CO 93. Take CO 93 north past Golden Gate Canyon Road, then travel 1.8 miles and take a left turn off of CO 93 onto West 56th Avenue (Pine Ridge Road). Continue about 1 mile until you see the trailhead parking lot on the right. CO 93 is a dangerous road; be cautious. Speed, blind spots, and wind play heavily in the accidents on CO 93.

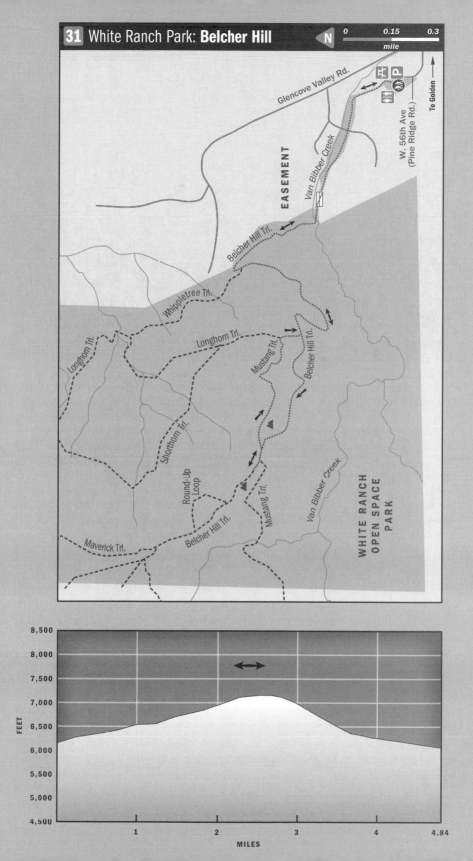

31 White Ranch Park: Belcher Hill

N

| 0 | 0.15 | 0.3 |
mile

To Golden

Glencove Valley Rd.

W. 56th Ave (Pine Ridge Rd.)

EASEMENT

Van Bibber Creek

Belcher Hill Trl.

Whippletree Trl.

Longhorn Trl.

Longhorn Trl.

Mustang Trl.

Belcher Hill Trl.

Shorthorn Trl.

Round-Up Loop

Van Bibber Creek

WHITE RANCH OPEN SPACE PARK

Mustang Trl.

Maverick Trl.

Belcher Hill Trl.

FEET

8,500
8,000
7,500
7,000
6,500
6,000
5,500
5,000
4,500

1   2   3   4   4.84

MILES

White Ranch Park has some of the most beautiful real estate outside of Denver. A spot like this would make a fine place to call home.

On your right is a part of the hogback that dominates the Front Range. To the left are new estates under construction. Cross an asphalt road and get right back on the trail. Do not turn and cross the cattle guard on the left. When you come to another gate, pass through, close the gate, and continue.

The trail crosses a footbridge and then curves to the left. Terrain changes quickly here because you enter a creek bed with trees, loose sand, exposed tree roots, and rocks. Large boulders skirt the trail. When I hiked, I dodged a lot of horse poop and a few frogs. In the early fall, the height of skunk cabbage has been said to determine the severity of winter in the Rocky Mountains. If this is the case, the six-foot cabbage we saw called for a long winter with deep snowdrifts.

The incline starts next, marked by a large fallen tree with an arm that protrudes out, almost a beacon to the trail. Since you are going up, the creek bed continues to fall down on your right. To the left is a wall of dirt covered by overgrown bushes. The trail is well maintained and characteristic of many of the Jefferson County Open Space trails: Volunteers tirelessly add erosion barriers such as landscaping logs that have been pushed into the sides of the trail. Barbed wire on the right side of the trail reminds us that the first part of the Belcher Hill Trail is part of an easement before it enters true open space.

Pass or pause at a bench to your left and then take the roundabout to the right. Foot travel can take either the stairs or the flat slats of wood designed for mountain bikes. Wind downward, cross a bridge over a creek, and then continue up and around the foothills. The trail at this point is red dirt, starts a steady uphill climb, and is wide enough for hikers to walk side by side.

Belcher Hill Trail is deceiving in spots. This nice flat section looks almost manageable.

The scenery here is comprised of custom-built estate homes. A large lake also comes into view. This is Ralston Reservoir, along with the Ralston Buttes. Bears and mountain lions have been spotted on this trail, but we only encountered black flies, chipmunks, and the sounds of crickets, airplanes, squirrels, and birds.

At the intersection of Longhorn Trail and Belcher Hill Trail, stay straight and do not go right. Views of Golden, Denver, and Table Mountain begin to peek out here. The incline is steady, although it does eventually relent. Exposure can be brutal on a sunny day without sunscreen. Continue up, up, up, until you reach the intersection of Belcher Hill Trail and Mustang Trail. In the shaded forest area of the trail, a bench awaits if you need a rest. Since you've reached the top of Belcher Hill, take a right on Mustang Trail and continue on a plateau that takes you through open meadow. As the trail starts its descent, a natural staircase is carved into the trail by tree roots and by man-made trail-erosion-prevention landscaping. This part of the loop is steep and full of large, loose rocks.

At the intersection of Longhorn Trail and Mustang Trail, turn right. Come out of the trees and begin a more gradual downhill, where you will soon encounter the intersection of Longhorn and Belcher Hill trails. Continue down and turn left on Belcher Hill Trail and back onto trail that you have already covered.

NEARBY ATTRACTIONS

Belcher Hill will encourage you to grab a trail map and explore the other trails in this 4,391-acre open space park. For further information, visit the Web site for Jefferson County Open Space: **jeffco.us/openspace**. Golden is home to the Colorado School of Mines and Coors Brewery.

North of Denver (Including Fort Collins and Rocky Mountain National Park)

N   0   3.5   7
miles

NORTH OF DENVER
(INCLUDING FORT COLLINS AND ROCKY MOUNTIAN NATIONAL PARK)

32 BUTTON ROCK PRESERVE: SLEEPY LION TRAIL

KEY AT-A-GLANCE INFORMATION

LENGTH: 5.5 miles

CONFIGURATION: Balloon

DIFFICULTY: Moderate

SCENERY: River, forest, meadow, waterfalls, dam, lake

EXPOSURE: Exposed along river and lake, shaded in forest

TRAFFIC: Moderate, but heavy in summer with climbers and anglers

TRAIL SURFACE: Hard-packed dirt, loose rocks

HIKING TIME: 3.5 hours

SEASON: All year

ACCESS: Free; open sunrise to sunset

MAPS: USGS Lyons

FACILITIES: Restrooms

SPECIAL COMMENTS: No bikes, dogs, horses, or swimming allowed. Wheelchair access to river views and wheelchair-accessible restroom.

IN BRIEF

Along the river and through the woods to a beautiful lake you go. This is an exceptional hike that pleases all the senses, from the thundering sound of water pouring from the dam to the sparkling ripples of the lake to the musky smell of shavings from the tree-thinning demonstration area. The variety of scenery, moderate pace, and longer length of this hike reward participants with a memorable outing.

DESCRIPTION

The trail begins at a white, metal fence that crosses a wide, dirt service road and allows only walk-in access. The trail is smooth, with a slight grade. Pass handicap-accessible viewing areas along the North Saint Vrain River (a popular spot for fly-fishing) and then Longmont Reservoir. Several rock walls that line the spillway are popular with rock climbers; appropriate gear is required for this activity.

Pass signs to Button Rock Dam and turn left onto Sleepy Lion Trail. The trail, which is covered in loose rocks and shaded with dense pines, narrows and steepens. Begin to climb as if on a gym stair-stepping machine and watch for the hillside to the left, since the steady ascent has produced quite a drop-off. This

GPS Trailhead Coordinates

UTM Zone (WGS84) 13T

Easting 0470930

Northing 4452960

Latitude N 40.226563°

Longitude W 105.341690°

Directions ───────────────→

From Denver, take I-25 north to CO 66. Travel west through Longmont on CO 66 and then through Lyons. Take a right off of CO 66 at the dead-end stoplight in Lyons, and go west on CO 36 3.8 miles toward Estes Park. Look for Shelly's Cottage on the left. Turn left there onto a dirt road labeled CR 80. Travel 2.8 miles to the trailhead, which is marked by a white metal fence that creates a dead end in the road and marks the beginning of the trail.

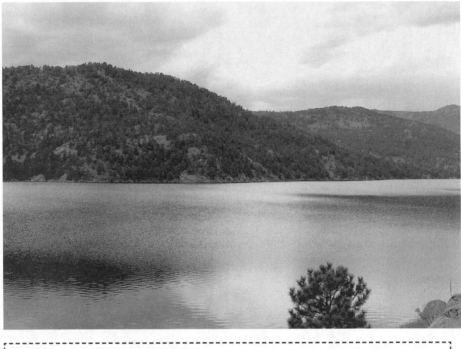

The cool waters of the Ralph Price Reservoir as seen after passing by the top of Button Rock Dam.

area has been appropriately nicknamed Deadman Gulch. The roar of the river is heard along the trail and quiets as the trail climbs. Continue until the trail reaches a plateau and opens to a beautiful meadow, complete with a view of Rocky Mountain National Park and the comfortable sounds of a babbling brook, a light breeze through dried grass, and crickets. From here, ascend another hill and watch for the universal hiking signs (a block human with a hiking stick and legs in stride) scattered around to guide the way.

As they say, what goes up must go down, and at a significantly rocky portion of the trail, it begins to descend. Flecks of mica, moss-covered boulders, and a cool, wet, vanilla smell coming from the dense pines and junipers dominate the trail.

At the intersection of Sleepy Lion Trail and Hall Ranch Open Space, continue to the right. (We are still in Button Rock Preserve.) The reservoir is in view, but pay attention to the directional arrows on the signs. At first it looks as if you should head straight for the water, but trust the signs that take you uphill through the rocks. The trail goes to the right, passing an iron gate on the left. Oddly enough, this part of the trail now contains smatterings of asphalt. The trail ascends and crosses live creeks teeming with water bugs. Aspen trees line the way and are beautiful when turning golden in early fall.

At the base of the Ralph Price Reservoir is the steep wall of Button Rock Dam, where a large amount of water shoots out of a culvert and into the river. Pass this on the right, turn toward the dam, and start up the "bonus trail" to the

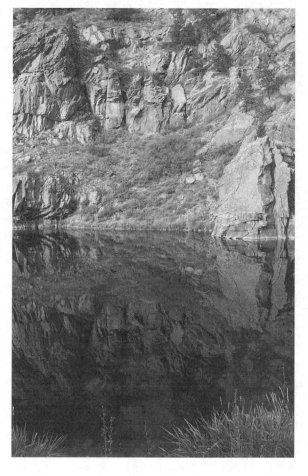

A still-life water portrait reflects the beauty along Sleepy Lion Trail.

right side of the dam wall. It takes hikers straight to the top of the dam wall and to the reservoir. Continue on the service road that winds around the right side of the lake. The water in the reservoir ranges from 60 to 100 feet in depth.

During the 1950s, Longmont was shifting from a highly agricultural town to a more technologically oriented economy. Mayor Ralph Price decided to build the Button Rock Dam over the North Saint Vrain River, just 7 miles upstream from Lyons. When a flood swept through the town, the dam saved Longmont from disaster. The flood filled the reservoir overnight instead of taking the projected years to fill.

When the service road forks, take a right. Continue past the ranger residence and through the tree-thinning demonstration area. A sign reads, "Learn how to Chip, Pile, Lop, and Scatter." Turn right at the intersection of Ralph Price Reservoir and Ralph Price Reservoir North Shore Line. Pass a restroom on the right, and turn left to continue down the service road. Pass the original turnoff for Sleepy Lion Trail and another restroom, and head back to the parking area.

NEARBY ATTRACTIONS

The Golden Ponds Natural Open Space boasts 94 acres of nature walkways, bikeways, ponds, and open space perfect for picnics, fishing, and wildlife observation. The park is located at Third Avenue and Hover Road in Longmont.

For more information, visit the Web site for the city of Longmont: **ci.longmont.co.us**.

33 CATHY FROMME PRAIRIE: FOSSIL CREEK TRAIL

KEY AT-A-GLANCE INFORMATION

LENGTH: 4.8 miles

CONFIGURATION: Out-and-back

DIFFICULTY: Easy

SCENERY: Meadow, views of Horsetooth Rock

EXPOSURE: Very exposed

TRAFFIC: Moderate

TRAIL SURFACE: Concrete

HIKING TIME: 2.5 hours

SEASON: All year

ACCESS: Free; open 5 a.m.–11 p.m.

MAPS: USGS Fort Collins

FACILITIES: Kiosk; restroom located just before Taft Hill Road

SPECIAL COMMENTS: Beware of the snakes, especially the Western rattlesnake, sunning themselves on the concrete. Rangers ask that hikers refrain from reaching into burrows along the trail, since rattlesnakes and black widow spiders live there. Stay on the trail and keep pets leashed. The rattlesnakes and birds of prey would much rather eat the abundant prairie dogs.

IN BRIEF

Cathy Fromme Prairie Natural Area, tagged as the jewel of the high plains, is an excellent and rare example of how the Colorado Front Range looked before it was settled. The rolling terrain, wetlands, and grasslands support a variety of plants and animals. Cathy Fromme, who passed away in 1992, was a local advocate for citizen involvement and environmental protection. She served on the Fort Collins City Council in 1991 and 1992.

DESCRIPTION

After leaving the parking area, turn right onto Fossil Creek Trail. Walk along the paved trail, adjacent to tall prairie grasses and weeds. Pass through an open gate and head left, down into the prairie. Pass an intersection of the trail from a residential area on the right. Continue left and travel through native shortgrass species that include buffalo grass, blue grama, little bluestem, needle and thread, and sideoats grama. Short information displays along the trail discuss various aspects of the prairie. Replicated animal tracks are also pressed into the pavement at regular intervals.

Pass a spur off the trail that leads to a memorial plaque and bench. You see an abundance of signs that warn of rattlesnakes, which tend to draw your attention to the

GPS Trailhead Coordinates

UTM Zone (WGS84) 13T

Easting 0491870

Northing 4484340

Latitude N 40.509737°

Longitude W 105.095961°

Directions ⟶

From Denver, take I-25 north to the Harmony Road exit in Fort Collins. Travel west on Harmony Road through Fort Collins; cross over College Avenue, and continue to Shields Street. Turn left and travel about 1 mile, where a parking sign directs you to the trailhead on the right.

0   0.2   0.4
mile

To downtown Fort Collins

68

Harmony Rd.

CR 17   Shields St.

Fossil Creek

P

Fossil Creek

Fromme Prairie Way

Fossil Creek Trl.

68

CR 19   Taft Hill Rd.

CATHY FROMME PRAIRIE

68

To Horsetooth Reservoir and Horsetooth Mountain Park

8,500

8,000

7,500

7,000

6,500

6,000

5,500

5,000

4,500

FEET

0.5   1   1.5   2   2.4

MILES

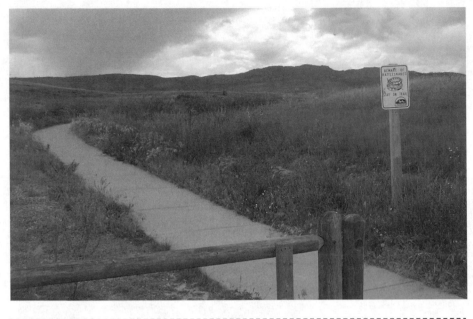

Signs warning hikers of rattlesnakes that frequent the area line the edge of the Fossil Creek Trail.

ground. Instead, all eyes should be on the views of Horsetooth Rock ahead. To the right is a new residential area and to the left is the prairie.

The trail, which started at a slight descent, now travels at a very slight ascent. It appears as if the entire trail will be rolling back and forth. Pass another spur that looks as if it leads to a residential area. When you pass a small rest area, continue toward Taft Hill Road. Cross over a bridge and the trail's namesake, Fossil Creek. Travel past another spur in the trail that goes to a restroom. Right after the spur for the restroom, go through an underpass with Taft Hill Road above you. Pass a sign that declares GREAT RAPTOR WATCHING. Birds of prey perch on trees, poles, benches, or fence posts: Red tail hawks and golden eagles are just two birds sighted on my afternoon hike. An observation building just beyond the opposite side of the trailhead is a good place to bring binoculars and identify these birds. Interactive displays discuss the relationship between raptors and their prey.

The Larimer County Landfill is to the left, but it's far enough away to prevent a distraction from the hike. Pass a spur on the right that goes through a neighborhood. Pass a private property sign and a gate. Cross over a bridge and stop at the end of the concrete. This is the end of the trail and our turnaround point.

NEARBY ATTRACTIONS

Other Fort Collins natural areas: **fcgov.com/naturalareas**. Horsetooth Mountain Open Space (**larimer.org/naturalresources**) and Lory State Park are nearby (**parks. state.co.us**).

GLEN HAVEN: CROSIER MOUNTAIN TRAIL 34

IN BRIEF

Crosier Mountain Trail is near the mountain town of Glen Haven. It's a cute little place and a miniature of neighboring Estes Park, with one bed-and-breakfast, one general store, one great gift shop, and a real estate office. Crosier Mountain is a small version of the massive trails that dominate neighboring Rocky Mountain National Park. It's a great workout with spectacular views and smaller crowds than are found in Estes Park.

DESCRIPTION

From the Rainbow Pit (gravel pit) trailhead for Crosier Mountain, leave the parking lot and the hillside that is eroding nearby. Pass through a wood gate. At first the trail is eroding, with large cracks and gullies formed by water. The path narrows and ascends at a steady incline through a forest of evergreen and aspen trees. Continue up and navigate the loose gravel and rocks.

Take the large switchback to the right and continue. You can still hear the noise from CR 43 here. The trail levels out for a short distance and then switchbacks again to begin a new ascent. Views from the trail open up to the left as trees thin out and meadows appear. Travel into low bushes and scattered trees on the packed-dirt path with exposed tree roots and scattered rocks.

KEY AT-A-GLANCE INFORMATION

LENGTH: 8 miles
CONFIGURATION: Out-and-back
DIFFICULTY: Difficult
SCENERY: Views of Estes Park, Rocky Mountain National Park; forested, meadows
EXPOSURE: Mostly shaded
TRAFFIC: Moderate
TRAIL SURFACE: Hard-packed dirt
HIKING TIME: 4 hours
SEASON: All year
ACCESS: Free; open sunrise to sunset
MAPS: USGS Glen Haven
FACILITIES: Trailhead kiosk
SPECIAL COMMENTS: Dogs must be leashed. Signs warn that this is bear country and ask hikers to stay on the trail.

GPS Trailhead Coordinates

UTM Zone (WGS84)   13T
Easting   0463940
Northing   4478350
Latitude   N 40.455031°
Longitude   W 105.425283°

Directions

From Denver, take I-25 north to US 34 west through Loveland. Travel to Drake, continuing on US 34; turn right onto CR 43. Pass the Garden Gate trailhead at 2.2 miles, and at 5.5 miles, reach the Rainbow Pit trailhead on the left. A large gravel pit cuts the south side of the road.

N

0   0.2   0.4
mile

To
Drake

CR 51B

CR 43

Rainbow
Pit

P

N. Fork Big Thompson River

CR 43

To
Glen Haven

Coyote
Rock

Piper
Meadows

ROOSEVELT
NATIONAL FOREST

The Road

Crosier
Mtn.

9,500

9,000

8,500

8,000

7,500

7,000

6,500

6,000

5,500

FEET

1   2   3   4

MILES

Views of Rocky Mountain National Park from the Crosier Mountain summit.

Continue through a series of switchbacks and walk over rose quartz that now dots the trail. Look across the valley to views of mountainsides lined with homes. Rose quartz, fool's gold, and loose rock now make up the trail. Trees provide a nice canopy in this early section. Other trailheads leading to Crosier Mountain are widely exposed and very hot in the summer months.

The trail levels out, descends for a section, and then rises again. Cross over a small gully; the trail levels out one more time and then makes a quick switchback. You see your first views of Rocky Mountain National Park from here. The trail is again eroded and very steep. As you cross the ridge, you'll see more views of Drake and the Big Thompson Canyon. The trail levels out again, passes boulder formations, and then descends for a while. Pass through a short lip and then travel up. The trail is wide here and a little overgrown in spots. Pass a sign to the left marking Coyote Rock.

At the intersection of Crosier Mountain, Glen Haven, and The Road, turn left. This route originates from The Road. After the turn, head down into a cool, small gully, then back up again. If legs and lungs are a little tired here, be assured that the intersection has marked the halfway point to the summit. The trail widens a little and enters a forest of lodgepole pines, where it levels out fairly well and provides a nice respite. But just as quickly, the trail goes back into rougher terrain, with rocks and loose gravel.

Hiking buddies Suellen May and Wyatt Lymber descend into a meadow along Crosier Mountain Trail.

At the intersection of Crosier Mountain, North Fork of the Big Thompson, and Glen Haven, turn right. The trail is steep and tiring from this point on. Social trails spur off the main trail, so keep to the left when there is a right turn-off. The trail finally levels out and travels through a small meadow with views of Longs Peak straight ahead, behind the dead trees. At the top of Crosier Mountain, the trail ends. The summit is character-ized by a large drop-off and views of Estes Park and Rocky Mountain National Park. Rest on the welcoming, large boulders, and then turn around to start the long walk back to the trailhead.

NEARBY ATTRACTIONS

Miller Fork, Storm Mountain, and West Creek trails (Canyon Lakes Ranger District): **fs.fed.us/arnf**. Estes Park and Rocky Mountain National Park: Estes Park Convention & Visitors Bureau (**estesparkcvb.com**) or Rocky Mountain National Park (**nps.gov/romo**).

HORSETOOTH MOUNTAIN OPEN SPACE:
HORSETOOTH FALLS AND HORSETOOTH ROCK

IN BRIEF

Horsetooth Rock is an important Front Range landmark and is affectionately known as the Tooth to locals. This trail combines a short walk through wildflowers to Horsetooth Falls, with a longer hike through dense forest to Horsetooth Rock.

DESCRIPTION

The trailhead is a confusing mix of mountain bike and foot traffic, so be careful to pass the service road and miscellaneous gates and go right on the Soderburg Trail. Be sure to carry a map of Horsetooth Mountain Open Space trails because the trails, albeit well marked, can be tricky to navigate.

The dirt trail, flanked on each side by seasonal wildflowers, starts with a slight grade but soon flattens and offers a view of CR 38. Trail workers have put a lot of loving care into this trail and placed flat rocks flush with the path. They act as walking stones on a part of the trail that becomes muddy in times of rain or runoff.

At the intersection of Soderburg Trail and Horsetooth Falls Trail, take a right. Crest the hill and take in views of Fort Collins homes and buildings, along with the neighboring meadow landscape that is brown and arid in

KEY AT-A-GLANCE INFORMATION

LENGTH: 7.2 miles
CONFIGURATION: Loop
DIFFICULTY: Moderate
SCENERY: Open meadow, forest; views of Horsetooth Reservoir and Fort Collins
EXPOSURE: Mostly shaded
TRAFFIC: Heavy near Horsetooth Falls; moderate around Horsetooth Rock
TRAIL SURFACE: Dirt, loose rocks
HIKING TIME: 4 hours
SEASON: All year
ACCESS: $6 (exact change required); open sunrise to sunset
MAPS: At trailhead; USGS Horsetooth Reservoir
FACILITIES: Restroom, water, emergency call box, information kiosk, picnic table under shelter, grill
SPECIAL COMMENTS: Some rock scrambling is required to get to the top of Horsetooth Rock. Larimer County Parks and Open Lands Department offers a pass ($65 resident, $85 nonresident; $10 disabled), which is available for the calendar year.

Directions

From Denver, take I-25 north to the Fort Collins/Harmony Road exit. Go left, traveling west on Harmony Road through Fort Collins until Harmony Road turns into CR 38E after the intersection with Taft Hill Road. Continue around the south end of Horsetooth Reservoir. Look for signs to Horsetooth Mountain Open Space and turn right into the parking lot.

GPS Trailhead Coordinates

UTM Zone (WGS84) 13T

Easting 0484700

Northing 4448720

Latitude N 40.522069°

Longitude W 105.180624°

N

0   0.2   0.4
mile

HORSETOOTH
MOUNTAIN
OPEN SPACE

Spring Creek Trl.

Towers Rd.

Westridge Trl.

Wathren Trl.

Herrington Trl.

Stout Trl.

Towers Rd.

Horsetooth
Rock

Audra Culver Trl.

Horsetooth Rock Trl.

Soderberg Trl.

Spring Creek Trl.

Stout Trl.

Horsetooth
Falls

service road

Soderburg Trl.

Horsetooth Falls Trl.

Spring Creek

service road

CR 38E

To
Fort Collins

Views of Horsetooth Reservoir from the trail to Horsetooth Falls and Horsetooth Rock.

fall and green and lush in spring. The trail ascends and is fairly exposed to the elements. A small bench off of the trail offers hikers a small respite. Descend through scattered pine trees.

As the trail starts to ascend again, notice two large boulders to the right along a creek bed that is dry for most of the year. Cross a wooden footbridge and climb a set of man-made stairs.

Go straight at the intersection of Horsetooth Falls and Spring Creek Trail and locate Horsetooth Falls, which is only a few yards from the intersection. On the left, a trail sign indicates a side trail that leads to the falls, where granite cliffs tower over small pools. The Rocky Mountains are known for their finicky water supply, so the falls could be gushing or just trickling. There is always a guarantee of a small trickle of water from the spring for which Spring Creek is named. The cliffs' cool shadows and the allure of calming water make this a good resting place.

Return on the side trail, and turn left on Spring Creek Trail. Spring Creek runs along this serene portion of the trail, through intermittent forest and meadows. Continue on a series of steep switchbacks to an overlook with more views of the falls. From here, resume your forward course and use the man-made fence as your guide.

At the intersection of Spring Creek Trail and Soderburg Trail, turn left onto a wide, dirt service road that steadily climbs toward Horsetooth Rock. Look left for views of Horsetooth Reservoir, Fort Collins, the outskirts of Loveland, and, on a clear day, the northeastern plains.

At the sign for Horsetooth Rock, turn right off of Soderburg Trail and begin a steep climb. The narrow trail winds through ponderosa pines and granite outcrops. As the trail climbs to the summit, traverse solid slabs of pink granite. The

Horsetooth Falls may just be a trickle (as shown here) or a gushing water feature, but the variety will keep you coming back for more.

Tooth looms overhead. It is possible to ascend the rock by crossing below the landmark to its north side, though the trip up requires a bit of nontechnical rock scrambling. Views of the Bellevue Valley appear as you pass through gaps in the rock.

Horsetooth Rock looks just as it sounds, like a horse's tooth—one large molar. According to Arapaho legend, the Tooth is the heart of the Great Red Warrior slain by the Great Black Warrior in a long and ferocious battle in the sky. The blood shed in the battle is said to have colored the rimrock red.

From the Tooth, return along the summit trail and take a right onto Soderburg Trail. Look out for wildlife, since mule deer like to roam here. At a blind corner on the Soderburg Trail, take the left route that directs hikers down the trail. Mountain bikers are asked to go right, down the service road. A bench is also available for a rest. The Soderburg Trail continues to a T intersection. Make a sharp right and follow the switchbacks back to the parking lot.

NEARBY ATTRACTIONS

Horsetooth Mountain Open Space is a 2,772-acre park and open space located in the foothills of Fort Collins with 28 miles of trails for hiking, mountain biking, and horseback riding. Horsetooth Reservoir offers boating, waterskiing, and fishing. For further information on more outdoor activities in the area, visit Larimer County Parks and Open Lands Department's Web site at **larimer.org/ naturalresources.**

LARIMER COUNTY: DEVIL'S BACKBONE TRAIL 36

IN BRIEF

The Devil's Backbone is a small section of the hogbacks found up and down the Front Range. The hogbacks are remnants of an ancient exposed seafloor that has been honed by the elements over thousands of years. It's an easy, well-maintained trail right outside of Loveland on the way to Estes Park (Rocky Mountain National Park).

DESCRIPTION

Start the hike by passing a large group of cottonwood trees, and take a quick break here if you need to use the shelter of the trees and the picnic tables scattered throughout. At this point, the trail is smooth, hard-packed red dirt flanked by landscape rocks.

The hogback in view may be seen from many different vantage points throughout the area and is more ancient than the Rocky Mountains. That is one reason that the folks at

---

Directions

From Denver, take I-25 north to CO 34 west toward Loveland and Estes Park (Rocky Mountain National Park). Still on CO 34, travel through Loveland (CO 34 is also known as West Eisenhower Boulevard in Loveland city limits), past Lake Loveland, and past all the shopping and strip malls and grocery stores. When you reach the western outskirts of town, you'll recognize the Devil's Backbone to the north of CO 34. Look for Hidden Valley Drive near the old water tank and for signs that mark Devil's Backbone. Turn right onto a good gravel road, which is Hidden Valley Drive. Trailhead parking is a half mile up the road on the left and marked by a beautiful metal sign that mimics the Backbone.

KEY AT-A-GLANCE INFORMATION

LENGTH: 3.48 miles

CONFIGURATION: Balloon

DIFFICULTY: Easy

SCENERY: Severe rock outcrop (hogback) that makes up Devil's Backbone, meadows, scrub bushes, raptor habitat, views of Rocky Mountains

EXPOSURE: No shade except for a few trees just beyond the trailhead

TRAFFIC: Heavy

TRAIL SURFACE: Dirt

HIKING TIME: 2 hours

SEASON: All year. Check with Larimer County Parks and Open Lands (larimer.org/parks) for seasonal trail closures for nesting birds.

ACCESS: Free, donation suggested at trailhead; open sunrise to sunset

MAPS: Open Space Trail Guide at trailhead; USGS Masonville

FACILITIES: Restroom, doggy pickup bags, picnic area, emergency call box

SPECIAL COMMENTS: We suggest hiking here on a weekday— perhaps as a beginning or an end to a trip up the Big Thompson Canyon. Dogs must be leashed. Do not climb on the rock formations. If no parking is available at trailhead, a sign suggests coming back later to reduce overuse.

GPS Trailhead Coordinates

UTM Zone (WGS84)   13T

Easting   0487500

Northing   4472900

Latitude   N 40.406619°

Longitude   W 105.147317°

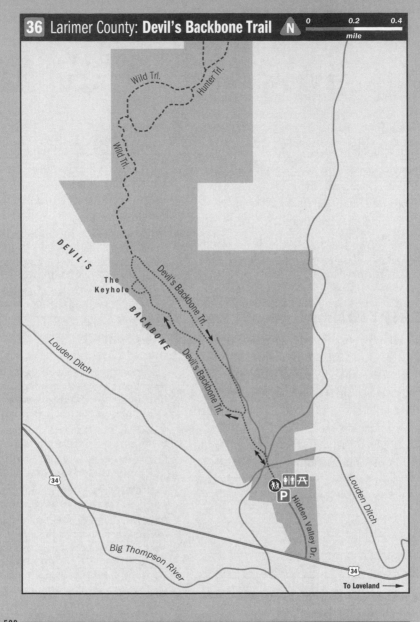

N

0   0.2   0.4

mile

Wild Trl.

Hunter Trl.

Wild Trl.

D E V I L ' S

The
Keyhole

B A C K B O N E

Devil's Backbone Trl.

Devil's Backbone Trl.

Louden Ditch

34

Louden Ditch

Hidden Valley Dr.

Big Thompson River

34

To Loveland →

8,500

8,000

7,500

7,000

6,500

6,000

5,500

5,000

4,500

FEET

0.5   1   1.5   2   2.5   3   3.48

MILES

A small peek of Devil's Backbone from the shaded portion at the beginning of the trail.

the Larimer County Parks and Open Lands ask that you do not climb on the fragile rock formations.

Pass an old mine shaft and Louden Ditch, an irrigation ditch circa 1878 that originally watered 12,000 acres of farmland. They are both fenced off and posted as private property.

This trail is shared by many mountain bikers, so the signs along the trail ask riders to take different routes than hikers. Other signs on the trail are single numbers that correlate with an interpretive brochure published by Larimer County Parks and Open Lands and available at the trailhead. These numbered markers point out areas of natural and historical interest from bird habitats to dinosaur fossil discoveries.

A staircase early in the trail is designed for foot traffic, so continue up the staircase and across the footbridge. Be very cautious on these wooden pieces of stair and bridge. While hiking the trail with my friend Shannon in a pelting rain of ice, I fell on the slick staircase. A second footbridge goes over a streambed that's dry in the fall but full of water in the spring.

A subdivision is going up to the east of the trail, and sounds of construction often echo off the hogback. Focus on the beauty of the area and the sounds of the many raptors and other birds that nest in the cavities of the Backbone. Red-tailed hawks, prairie falcons, golden eagles, ravens, and a colony of swallows all make their homes here.

Turn left at the first trail bench and continue as the trail gradually ascends to the base of the Backbone. From a marked overlook, take in incredible views of the Backbone and the Rocky Mountains. The overlook is a small detour to the left of the trail; take it and come right back to the main path. Again, views are nice, despite development on the west side of the Backbone.

In the 1800s, hops cultivator Alfred Wild bought the southern portion of the Devil's Backbone. Wild is noted as one of the area's pioneer industrialists. Larimer County bought the Backbone in 1998 opened it to the public in 1999.

Cross a large piece of rock in the trail and pass the signpost labeled "5." This gray rock, which is part of the Morrison Formation, dates back approximately 150 million years. Dinosaur bones and footprints have been found in the Morrison Formation all along the Front Range, but none are visible from this trail. A prehistoric elephant and a jawbone with seven teeth were discovered in a nearby gypsum mine.

Follow the trail to Keyhole Bypass, a special window carved directly through the Backbone. The Keyhole was formed by erosion of coarse-grained rocks and is only one of the geological attractions of this hike. The region that the trail traverses is so rich in geological interest—with rock outcrops from the Morrison, Entrada, and Triassic Lykins Formations—that local fourth graders often visit the trail to study geology.

Turn back around and continue north on the main trail to the Backbone Trail and Wild Trail intersection. You have been on a foot-traffic-only section of the trail (along the eastern ridge of the Backbone) until this point, but will go back on the multiuse trail back to the trailhead. This gives you the opportunity to complete a perfect loop and experience different vantage points of the Backbone. To do this, take a right at this intersection. Many bikers continue on to the left at this point and add another 7 miles to the route.

The vistas of the Backbone drop down to a lower level, where views of the area mountains are limited. However, a sunset hike rewards you with an amazing light show: mahogany-colored brush hills, purple alpenglow sky, and a fiery red hue along the hogback, which may be attributed to the Backbone's namesake. The loop reconnects at the footbridge. Continue down the stairs, across to the trees, and back home again. A donation box at the trailhead benefits Larimer County Parks and Open Lands. For good karma's sake, we deposited $5.

NEARBY ATTRACTIONS

Big Thompson Canyon and the Dam Store are a short drive west of the trailhead. Loveland has commendable shopping, dining, and lodging. A cute bed-and-breakfast, Wild Lane Inn, is less than 1 mile from the trailhead. Loveland is famous for its sculpture artists, the annual Sculpture in the Park, and the Loveland Valentine program, which re-mails Valentines from Loveland to the intended destinations.

For further information, visit the Web site for Larimer County Parks and Open Lands: **larimer.org/naturalresources.**

LARIMER COUNTY: KRUGER ROCK

IN BRIEF

Kruger Rock Trail is located in Larimer County's Hermit Park Open Space. Hermit Park, about 2 miles southeast of Estes Park, is relatively new (it opened in 2008). This hike is easy to find and a good lung buster. With an elevation gain of more than 900 feet and scenery that is just as aggressive, you have a well-rounded hike. Much of the trail offers a rarely seen perspective of Rocky Mountain National Park, and the views alone are worth the trip.

DESCRIPTION

Pass through the parking lot and head toward the pavilion, picnic tables, restrooms, and horseshoe pits. Cross through the trees via a short path. Protected wetlands and fields surround the trailhead area on either side.

Cross the main road and travel to the main Kruger Rock trailhead. The trail climbs gradually up an open hillside and passes through a small meadow dotted with wildflowers in the summer. Fireweed, Indian paintbrushes, and aspen trees are plentiful. Continue in this direction at a slight incline. The aspen trees become dense as you pass a large rock outcrop to the left of the trail.

Turning to the north, you will come to the first switchback of the trail, taking you through a boulder field where the first elevated views of

KEY AT-A-GLANCE INFORMATION

LENGTH: 3.8 miles

CONFIGURATION: Out-and-back

DIFFICULTY: Moderate

SCENERY: Meadow, forest; views of Estes Park, Rocky Mountain National Park, Mount Meeker, Longs Peak, Continental Divide, and Mummy Range

EXPOSURE: Sunny in meadow, shaded in areas with trees

TRAFFIC: Minimal

TRAIL SURFACE: Hard-packed dirt, loose rocks, some sandy spots

HIKING TIME: 2 hours

SEASON: All year (some portions may be icy during winter)

ACCESS: Pay $6 daily entrance fee per vehicle

MAPS: USGS Panorama Peak

FACILITIES: Restroom, picnic area, meeting pavilion, RV hookups, cabin rentals

SPECIAL COMMENTS: Dogs must be leashed. Reserve top-notch RV or tent campsites April–October at larimercamping.com or (800) 397-7795. Cabins are open and may be reserved all year. A camping permit is required for each campsite for each night in addition to entrance permits.

Directions

From Denver, take I-25 north to CO 66, and travel west on CO 66 for 16 miles to Lyons. Take a right off of CO 66 at the dead-end stoplight in Lyons, and go west on CO 36 for 16.7 miles. The entrance to Hermit Park is on the left. Take the dirt road to the Kruger Rock Trail parking area near the pavilion.

GPS Trailhead Coordinates

UTM Zone (WGS84) 13T

Easting 0458792

Northing 4465229

Latitude N 40.336586°

Longitude W 105.485147°

0   0.25   0.5
mile

N

To Lyons
36
To Estes Park

Hermit's Hollow Campground

Bobcat Campground

Homestead Meadows Connector Trl.

HERMIT PARK

P

Kruger Rock Trl.

Kruger Campground

Granite Gulch Campground

P

Kruger Rock

ROOSEVELT NATIONAL FOREST

10,500
10,000
9,500
9,000
8,500
8,000
7,500
7,000
6,500

FEET

0.5   1   1.5   1.9

MILES

Turtle Rock peeks out along the trail and greets Kruger Rock Trail visitors.

the Rocky Mountain National Park and Lake Estes can be seen. The switchbacks continue to ease the climb, and what comes up does come down, at least a little bit here and there, so expect some respite.

The first such break comes with a slight decline in the trail as it leads to a false summit, where the first views of the Mummy Range can be seen to the northwest. A short descent follows the ridge to the southwest, keeping the Mummy Range in view. The trail becomes sandy in small patches during the slight descent with rocky outcrops popping up throughout.

The trail eventually crosses back and forth over the ridge, keeping with the ascent, as Mummy Range comes in and out of view. The trail continues slightly downward until reaching another false summit that offers a 180-degree view of the park and the surrounding mountains. At this point the trail begins a steep climb as it switchbacks up the ascent. The trail eventually flattens out slightly as it leads southwest along the mountain. Longs Peak, Mount Meeker, and the Continental Divide are in the viewfinder.

The switchbacks continue up the mountain, and Kruger Rock comes in full view at another false summit. At this point, you can head back the way you came, or try some amateur rock climbing and head up Kruger Rock. Routes through the middle or around the west side of Kruger require a little scrambling up the rock.

NEARBY ATTRACTIONS

Estes Park: **estesparkcvb.com.** Rocky Mountain National Park: **nps.gov/romo.** Try other new trails or rent a cabin overnight at Hermit Park: **larimer.org/naturalresources.**

38 LORY STATE PARK: ARTHUR'S ROCK

KEY AT-A-GLANCE INFORMATION

LENGTH: 3.62 miles

CONFIGURATION: Out-and-back

DIFFICULTY: Difficult

SCENERY: Meadow, forest, views of Horsetooth Reservoir

EXPOSURE: Sunny in meadow, shaded in alpine portion

TRAFFIC: Moderate, only open to foot travel

TRAIL SURFACE: Hard-packed dirt, loose rocks

HIKING TIME: 2.5 hours

SEASON: All year

ACCESS: $6 per vehicle, $3 for individual; passes must be posted on windshield; daily pass is valid from the day purchased until noon the following day; open sunrise to sunset

MAPS: Lory State Park map at visitor center; USGS Horsetooth Reservoir

FACILITIES: Kiosk and restroom at trailhead; purchase park passes, learn about the park environment, view interpretive displays, and buy souvenirs at the visitor center

SPECIAL COMMENTS: This area is well patrolled, and park rules are strictly enforced. Look for rules in the Lory State Park map, at the trailhead, and at the visitor center. Controlled hunting is allowed.

GPS Trailhead Coordinates

UTM Zone (WGS84) 13T

Easting   0485260

Northing 4490200

Latitude N 40.562438°

Longitude W 105.174118°

IN BRIEF

Arthur's Rock, named for an early settler, is a granite outcrop in Lory State Park. At an elevation of 6,780 feet, summit hikers are rewarded with breathtaking views of Lory State Park, Horsetooth Reservoir, and the Fort Collins area. Arthur's Rock is a good, short hike for Fort Collins residents and an easy hike for someone in Denver who wants to spend the day in the Fort Collins area.

DESCRIPTION

Arthur's Rock Trail begins to the right of the restrooms and trailhead kiosk. Formerly ranchland, Lory State Park is a 2,400-acre parcel that was purchased in 1967 and named in honor of Charles Lory, president of Colorado State University in Fort Collins from 1909 to 1940. Lory's diverse terrain is home to mule deer, wild turkeys, black bears, mountain lions, coyotes, squirrels, cottontail rabbits, blue grouse, mourning doves, songbirds, and many reptiles.

Directions

From Denver, take I-25 north to the CO 14 exit in Fort Collins. Travel west through Fort Collins; CO 14 is also Mulberry Road in Fort Collins city limits. Turn right onto College Avenue/CO 287. Continue through northern Fort Collins toward La Porte. Do not take 287 toward Laramie; instead, continue on CR 54G. Follow signs to Lory State Park. Turn left on CR 52E at Vern's Restaurant and then turn left on CR 23 in Bellevue. Turn right on CR 25G, then left onto the gravel road (marked Lory State Park) that leads inside the park boundary. Pay at the visitor center and then drive to the very end of the road. The trailhead is visible from here.

0   0.2   0.4
mile

N

To
Fort Collins

Horsetooth Reservoir

Visitor
Center

Timber Trl.

Valley Trl.

Valley Trl.

Eltuck
Bay

Westridge Trl.

Well Gulch Nature Trl.

Eltuck
Picnic Area

Homestead
Picnic Area

Orchard
Cove

LORY
STATE PARK

Westridge Trl.

Arthur's
Rock

Arthur's Rock Trl.

Overlook Trl.

Valley Trl.

Valley Trl.

alternate trl.

meadow

Arthur's Rock Trl.

Shoreline Trl.

Mill Creek Trl.

8,500
8,000
7,500
7,000
6,500
6,000
5,500
5,000
4,500

FEET

0.5   1   1.5   1.81

MILES

Views from the top of Arthur's Rock are expansive. Here Horsetooth Reservoir is in the viewfinder.

The trail is characterized by rocks and smooth, hard-packed dirt. Cross two bridges and then head up Arthur's Rock gulch, a harrowing slot between rock cliffs. The path is narrow with boulder outcrops on both sides and well maintained with man-made staircases, natural staircases, and man-made bridges. The incline is steady with manageable switchbacks. The first views from the trail include a bit of the Horsetooth Reservoir and Lory State Park scenery, which includes unique rock outcrops, sandstone hogbacks, grassy open meadows, shrubby hillsides, and ponderosa pine forests.

If you're afraid of heights or are subject to vertigo, short portions at the beginning of this trail may trigger a minor sweat. After crossing the ridge and coming around from the switchbacks and views, the path lands you into an expansive meadow complete with a quaint bridge. Sunflowers grow tall in the late summer and early fall; grass sways back and forth at hip level. The gentle rocking is soothing as the meadow passes quickly and the first views of Arthur's Rock appear to the right. Until now, this massive rock structure has been hidden from view.

Pass a sign that marks Arthur's Rock Trail and Mill Creek Link Trail. Mill Creek Link Trail is a sharp left behind you, so continue straight on the Arthur's Rock Trail. Mill Creek Link Trail accesses Horsetooth Mountain Open Space. Many connector trails can be found throughout Horsetooth Mountain Open Space and Lory State Park.

Cottonwood trees line the creek that runs to your right, but soon the trail leaves the creek and enters a forest. Reach a sign that splits the trail and offers an

Arthur's Rock alternate route to the left and Arthur's Rock Trail straight ahead. Continue straight on Arthur's Rock Trail. This route takes you to the top of the massive, sun-kissed rock formation, but does so with many forgiving switchbacks. This trail has many signs, and the next one points to the summit of Arthur's Rock and a scenic overlook. Take a second to go off trail on a small footpath to the right and sneak a preview of the scenery. Back on the trail, come face to face with the vertical body of Arthur's Rock. Glowing red at dusk, this smooth, towering, vertical rock is at arm's length. The trail, with exposed roots and rocks, is wide enough at this point for one hiker.

Don't be alarmed if you hear voices on the trail. Arthur's Rock is massive and effectively echoes the faintest sounds. Go up, up, and up, and once your quads are in full burn, the trail levels. I promise. A lot of poison ivy grows along this trail, so please remember: "Leaves of three, let them be." Signs posted along the trail remind you of the poison ivy dangers. One park perk: Wildflowers, animals, and birds can all be studied with the aid of a guided hike available to groups by reservation.

At this point, you have ascended the south face of Arthur's Rock and are now ready for the remaining challenge of the trail, one major reason why I've rated this hike as difficult. Continuing, reach a small saddle on the hill and come to the intersection of Timber Trail and Arthur's Rock Summit. Bear right toward the summit. A sign here reads ROUTE TO SUMMIT, DIFFICULT TRAIL, USE CAUTION. A little bouldering is required here, so be prepared to turn back if you are not comfortable with scrambling over large rocks. No technical equipment is required, though, except the use of both hands and steady feet. Trail volunteers have obviously put many meticulous hours into this portion of the trail, making sure it is safe and easy to navigate. Move on to the summit and look to the east. The view pans from the waters of Horsetooth Reservoir to the trees and buildings of Fort Collins and then expands to the vast flatland of the Colorado prairie. Turn around and head back down again the way you came.

39 RABBIT MOUNTAIN: EAGLE WIND TRAIL

KEY AT-A-GLANCE INFORMATION

LENGTH: 3.9 miles

CONFIGURATION: Balloon

DIFFICULTY: Easy

SCENERY: Foothills, views of Continental Divide, cacti, prairie grasses, shrubs, short pines

EXPOSURE: Short-grass steppe environment; July and August are especially hot under the direct midday sun

TRAFFIC: Mild on weekdays

TRAIL SURFACE: Dirt

HIKING TIME: 2 hours

SEASON: All year

ACCESS: Free; open sunrise to sunset

MAPS: USGS Hygiene; maps at trailhead

FACILITIES: Restrooms, picnic facilities, and a group shelter that can accommodate 30 people

SPECIAL COMMENTS: Dogs must be leashed. The southeastern section of Rabbit Mountain is closed February 1–July 31 to protect wildlife during birthing and nursing season. Closures do not affect trail use, but visitors found in closed areas south and east of the Eagle Wind Trail are fined.

IN BRIEF

Rabbit Mountain is an excellent hike on an exposed plateau that offers views of the Colorado prairie and three amazing mountain ranges: Indian Peaks, Rocky Mountain National Park, and the Continental Divide. It's easy enough for families, yet interesting enough for seasoned hikers.

DESCRIPTION

From the parking area, veer left and then immediately head right at the first fork up the trail toward Eagle Wind Trail. The hard-packed dirt trail with loose rocks ascends slightly at first. Cut across the hill via trail switchbacks and take a right at the junction of Little Thompson Overlook Trail, Indian Mesa Trail, and Eagle Wind Trail. Prairie dogs and their burrows line the edges of the trail, and raptors are often seen flying overhead, scouting these dogs. Signs at the trailhead warn of rattlesnakes, since they are common around Rabbit Mountain and like to sun themselves on warm boulders and sunny slopes. Be aware of their possible presence.

Continue over the bridge that traverses the Saint Vrain Supply Canal and crosses the service road. Indian Mesa Trail runs parallel to this route for a few more yards. Head south

GPS Trailhead Coordinates

UTM Zone (WGS84) 13T

Easting   0480950

Northing   4454900

Latitude   N 40.244329°

Longitude   W 105.223973°

Directions

From Denver, take I-25 north to CO 66 exit. Turn left, traveling west on CO 66 through Longmont almost to the town of Lyons. Turn right on 53rd Street, which turns into 55th Street, and follow signs to Rabbit Mountain.

39 Rabbit Mountain: Eagle Wind Trail

N

0   0.2   0.4
mile

Little Thompson River

Little Thompson Overlook Trl.

St. Vrain Supply Canal

tunnel

Indian Mesa Trl.

To
Lyons

P

St. Vrain Supply Canal

Eagle Wind Trl.

RABBIT
MOUNTAIN

Eagle Wind Trl.

N. 55th St.

Rabbit
Mtn.

To
Longmont

8,500

8,000

7,500

7,000

6,500

6,000

5,500

5,000

4,500

FEET

1   2   3   3.9

MILES

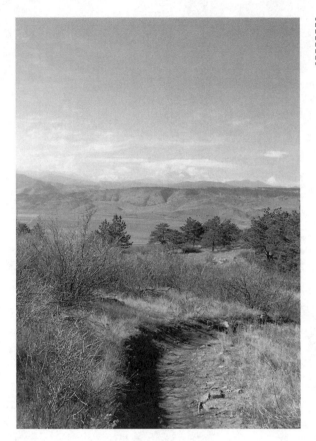

and pass a memorial bench on the left. This resting spot was appropriately picked because views of Mount Meeker and Longs Peak to the west are prevalent here. Views of civilization, such as homes and a gravel pit, can also be seen from here.

Rabbit Mountain is a transition zone, dividing the Saint Vrain drainage basin from the Big Thompson drainage basin. Geologists say that this area was once tropical lowland covered by rivers, swamps, and lagoons. Where hikers wander today, dinosaurs and other reptiles did their own wandering through lush vegetation. Historians also point out that Native Americans lived in this area for at least 5,000 years because of the abundant game, natural springs, and shelter from the strong west winds.

Eagle Wind Trail is a balloon, so hikers start the loop portion of this trail after approximately 1 mile of hiking. At an obvious split in the trail, take the left route. The nesting fine area mentioned before begins here, so be sure to stay on the trail at all times. Take in great views of Twin Peaks to the west and the plains to the northeast. Views of Rabbit Mountain to the east are obscured here by low-lying ponderosa pines, but not to worry since the mountain summit is not the final destination, nor is it accessible by this hike.

Modern-day trail trivia says that Jack Moomaw, the second owner of the Rabbit Mountain property, was Rocky Mountain National Park's first forest ranger. His family sold Rabbit Mountain to Boulder County in 1984, ensuring the preservation of the land in its natural state.

On the upper portion of this plateau, you may hear airplanes overhead, the chirping of prairie dogs, or the buzz of insects. Rabbit Mountain is an important winter feeding area for large herds of deer due to mild weather and plentiful prairie grasses. Deer also attract mountain lions, so it is not surprising that these large cats have been spotted here.

The trail enters a stand of fragrant ponderosa pines and continues through patches of cacti, yuccas, and tall prairie grasses. The trail is flat as it crosses the hill's plateau before it takes a wide turn and loops back to the right as it passes Rabbit Mountain on the left. The trail drops slightly and then climbs a short hill. Cut through a small open meadow, head through more ponderosa pines, and then hike back to the starting point of the loop. From this point, retrace your route back to the trailhead.

NEARBY ATTRACTIONS

Little Thompson Overlook Trail at Rabbit Mountain; Indian Mesa Trail. For more information: **bouldercounty.org/openspace.**

40 ROCKY MOUNTAIN NATIONAL PARK: GEM LAKE

KEY AT-A-GLANCE INFORMATION

LENGTH: 3.4 miles

CONFIGURATION: Out-and-back

DIFFICULTY: Moderate

SCENERY: Views of Estes Park, Rocky Mountain National Park, Twin Owls, alpine lake

EXPOSURE: Mostly shaded

TRAFFIC: Heavy

TRAIL SURFACE: Hard-packed dirt, some loose rocks and exposed tree roots

HIKING TIME: 2.5 hours

SEASON: All year

ACCESS: $20; open sunrise to sunset

MAPS: Estes Park Chamber of Commerce or Rocky Mountain National Park; USGS Estes Park

FACILITIES: Trailhead kiosk

SPECIAL COMMENTS: Dogs are not allowed here or on any trail in Rocky Mountain National Park. No horses, and no bikes. A backcountry permit is required for fires or overnight camping.

IN BRIEF

Gem Lake, if you'll pardon the pun, is a jewel. Located on the eastern edge of Rocky Mountain National Park, this trailhead is one of the closest to the town of Estes Park.

DESCRIPTION

To begin this hike, leave your car and walk to the trailhead and signs that mark the beginning of the Gem Lake Trail. Gem Lake's lower elevation in relation to the rest of Rocky Mountain National Park, along with the hike's southern exposure, makes this a great year-round hike. Estes Park is home to retirees, families, and other outdoors enthusiasts, so both the very old and very young frequent this trail.

In 2007, the Twin Owls and Gem Lake trailheads were combined and renamed the Lumpy Ridge trailhead. Until then, the trails split the crowds pretty evenly, so access to Gem Lake may be a little more crowded than usual. You're also hiking a trail that is 0.3 miles shorter than those I've featured in previous books.

In a few yards a steady climb begins, supplemented by short switchbacks that weave in and out of the trees and skirt around large rocks. After 0.5 miles, the Gem Lake Trail reaches a junction with the trail that leads west

GPS Trailhead Coordinates

UTM Zone (WGS84) 13T
Easting 0456920
Northing 4471410
Latitude N 40.392175°
Longitude W 105.507603°

Directions ⟶

From Denver, take I-25 north to US 34. Stay on US 34 until it intersects Big Thompson Avenue/Elkhorn Avenue and turns into Wonderview Avenue. Pass the Stanley Historic District and take the first right onto MacGregor Avenue. Follow MacGregor as it veers right and turns into Devils Gulch Road, and follow it until you reach the Lumpy Ridge trailhead turnoff on the left.

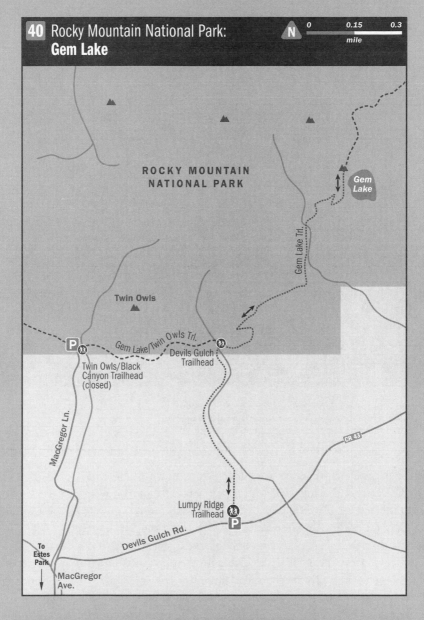

ROCKY MOUNTAIN
NATIONAL PARK

Gem Lake

Gem Lake Trl.

Twin Owls

Gem Lake|Twin Owls Trl.

Devils Gulch
Trailhead

Twin Owls/Black
Canyon Trailhead
(closed)

MacGregor Ln.

CR 43

Lumpy Ridge
Trailhead

To
Estes
Park

MacGregor
Ave.

Devils Gulch Rd.

N

0   0.15   0.3
mile

FEET

9,500
9,000
8,500
8,000
7,500
7,000
6,500
6,000
5,500

0.5   1   1.5   1.82

MILES

Twin Owls rock formation as seen from Gem Lake Trail.

to the Twin Owls—massive rock formations that resemble two giant owls resting on the crest of the hill. This intersection mostly marks access for rock climbers and their left turn to the owls, which you can see as you access the trailhead by car (a good point of reference is to look behind the Stanley Hotel). The climbing here is very technical, and climbers observe a strict code of conduct.

Staying on the Gem Lake Trail, turn right (east) and follow the trail as it climbs moderately. To the right, catch the first views of Rocky Mountain National Park and one of its more famous mountains: Longs Peak. A popular fourteener, or a peak 14,000 feet or higher, Longs can be found by looking for the silhouette of a beaver climbing up the side of a hill. The peak is at the beaver's nose.

Follow the sandy footpath near where heavy foot traffic has cut many random paths to scenic overlooks. Continue over smooth rock outcrops, and drink in the views of Lake Estes and Estes Park. The trail veers to the left and becomes even softer and sandier. On one of my hikes here, I saw a young racked buck, a rare sight this close to town.

Descend into a small, rocky canyon, where you find a bench and Paul Bunyan's Boot. Another rock formation of legend, this one resembles an oversize boot propped on its heel. (Note the hole in the sole.) Continue up the many switchbacks, passing a precariously placed outhouse along the way. This portion of the trail is quite narrow and navigates through a large boulder field and granite slabs.

The waters of Gem Lake may be cold, but her jewels sparkle in the sunlight.

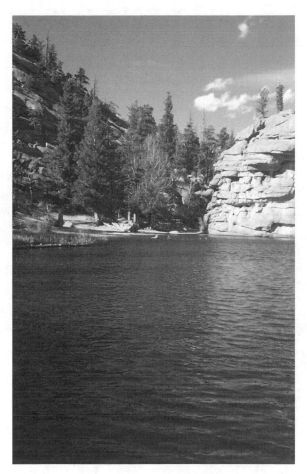

Gem Lake comes into view at the base of granite cliffs with boulders and a small beach at the water's edge. This mountain lake is a bit cold for the body, but a few minutes' respite here will cleanse the soul. When the sun hits the water, you'll see the mix of jewel tones—emerald, sapphire, ruby, and diamond—that gives the lake its name. To return to the trailhead, head back the way you came. If you have more time, plenty of hikes continue past Gem Lake and allow you to venture for hours, if not days, in Rocky Mountain National Park.

NEARBY ATTRACTIONS

The Stanley Historic District houses the famous Stanley Hotel, where Stephen King supposedly got his inspiration for *The Shining*. It's fun to walk around the hotel, and the food is excellent. Estes Park has a nice mix of shopping, dining, historic attractions, and lodging. Rocky Mountain National Park is a treasure that offers hiking, picnicking, camping, fishing, rock climbing, snowshoeing, cross-country skiing, birding, and photography in the 74 mountain peaks that reach elevations of at least 14,000 feet.

For further information, visit the Web sites for Estes Park Convention & Visitors Bureau (**estesparkcvb.com**) or Rocky Mountain National Park (National Park Service) (**nps.gov/romo**).

41 ROCKY MOUNTAIN NATIONAL PARK: LILY MOUNTAIN

KEY AT-A-GLANCE INFORMATION

LENGTH: 3.92 miles

CONFIGURATION: Out-and-back

DIFFICULTY: Moderate

SCENERY: Alpine, views of Estes Park and Rocky Mountain National Park

EXPOSURE: Mostly shaded

TRAFFIC: Moderate

TRAIL SURFACE: Dirt, loose rock

HIKING TIME: 2.5 hours

SEASON: April–October

ACCESS: $20; open sunrise to sunset

MAPS: USGS Longs Peak

FACILITIES: Call box

SPECIAL COMMENTS: No facilities here; parking is limited. Dogs are now OK on this trail.

IN BRIEF

Lily Mountain is ideal for visitors who don't have the time or money to hike Rocky Mountain National Park. Lily Mountain, a classic alpine hike with rewarding views and a steady climb, is often passed over for other hikes in the vicinity, such as Twin Sisters, and the hike is often confused with the small walk around Lily Lake. It is one of the least crowded near Estes Park.

DESCRIPTION

Leave the parking area and begin to climb directly from the trailhead. Pass a National Park Service boundary post and a Lily Mountain sign. The first half mile parallels CO 7 as the trail begins its ascent along the ridge. Large pines and boulder clusters dominate the landscape here. The hard-packed dirt trail has loose rocks and some exposed tree roots. Expect snow on the trail if you hike outside of the recommended seasons. We hiked in early winter and encountered packed snow from the trailhead on.

Early in the trail the landscape also includes aspen trees and consistent light filtering through the trees. The trail takes an uncharacteristic dip, then flattens out before ascending a small

GPS Trailhead Coordinates

UTM Zone (WGS84) 13T

Easting   0454560

Northing   4462470

Latitude   N 40.311511°

Longitude   W 105.534772°

Directions

From Denver, take I-25 north to CO 66. Travel west through Longmont on CO 66 and then through Lyons. Take a right at the dead-end stoplight in Lyons and go west on CO 36 to Estes Park. Turn left off of CO 36 onto CO 7 before the first stoplight in Estes Park. Go south on CO 7, past Mary's Lake. The road curves sharply. After 5.7 miles from the turn onto CO 7, look for a small parking area on the right shoulder of the road and the Lily Mountain trail marker.

N

0   0.2   0.4
mile

To
Estes Park
and 34 36

7

ROOSEVELT
NATIONAL FOREST

S. Vrain Ave.

big
rock

7

Fish Creek

Aspen Brook

Lily Mtn.

ROCKY MOUNTAIN
NATIONAL PARK

S. Vrain Ave.

P

7

Lily Lake

P

10,000
9,500
9,000
8,500
8,000
7,500
7,000
6,500
6,000

FEET

0.5   1   1.5   1.96
MILES

The views from the top of Lily Mountain are amazing—Rocky Mountain National Park and her valleys with snow-capped peaks.

man-made staircase and starting a series of small switchbacks. As the trail crests, the Estes Park Valley, Mary's Lake, and the town of Estes Park come into view. Pass a natural break in the trail that has been carved by hikers going off of the trail to the right and continue to the left. This boulder-shaded spot is a nice place for a rest. From this junction, start another gradual climb toward Lily Mountain. The summit is not yet in view. Continue on the trail and pass more large rocks and a picturesque dead tree that stands as a sentinel on the right after a large switchback.

At a large outcrop of boulders, you'll see an overlook on the right. Look to the left for views of Rocky Mountain National Park and right for more views of the Estes Park Valley and the town of Estes Park. Get back on the trail and continue to climb. The trail becomes dark and shaded, with large pine trees clustered together.

As the trail continues to ascend with switchbacks, built-in erosion control devices, mainly logs and landscaping materials, are along the path. This side of the ridge can be very windy, and you will hear the sounds of the highway far below.

Pass a trail marker at the crest of the hill. Continue to the right toward Lily Mountain's Peak, which consists of a large rock pile. Cairns mark the route to the top, and hikers must scramble up this last part of the trail. Views from the top are extraordinary and include Longs Peak, Twin Sisters, and the Mummy Range. After photographs, maybe lunch, and a rest, turn around to retrace the same route.

NEARBY ATTRACTIONS

Rocky Mountain National Park hikes: **estesparkcvb.com** or **nps.gov/romo**.

ROCKY MOUNTAIN NATIONAL PARK: LONGS PEAK   42

IN BRIEF

The excursion up this awe-inspiring mountain blurs the lines between a hike and a climb. The 15 miles will likely rank among the most spectacular yet hard-earned miles you have ever hiked. This mountain displays both imposing stature and magnificent beauty that validate its popularity. Longs Peak is the tallest mountain in Rocky Mountain National Park and the fourteener that sits farthest north in Colorado. It is also the easternmost point of the Continental Divide.

DESCRIPTION

Leave the trailhead and follow the East Longs Peak Trail (Keyhole Route) and begin an enchanting jaunt through the trees. Pass a small campground named Goblins Forest. At 1.9 miles, reach a well-constructed bridge crossing over a small cascading waterfall. This is a beautiful place to take a break.

Your first views of Longs Peak are here as the trees transition to shorter vegetation. At 2.5 miles, a fork appears in the trail. Follow the sign left toward the summit. After another mile, you'll reach the junction of the Chasm Lake Trail. This is another great spot to rest, as there is a pit toilet and a vista of the east Diamond

KEY AT-A-GLANCE INFORMATION

LENGTH: 15 miles
CONFIGURATION: Out-and-back
DIFFICULTY: Difficult
SCENERY: Evergreen forest, spectacular mountain views, tundra
EXPOSURE: Shaded at beginning, no shade at end, high alpine exposure
TRAFFIC: Heavy
TRAIL SURFACE: Dirt, loose rock, talus, large boulders, large flat slate
HIKING TIME: 12 hours
SEASON: June–October
ACCESS: $20; open sunrise to sunset
MAPS: USGS Longs Peak
FACILITIES: Ranger station with ranger usually on duty, restrooms, camping sites, and picnic facilities; museum, plentiful information on hikes and Rocky Mountain National Park
SPECIAL COMMENTS: Dogs are not allowed on any trail in Rocky Mountain National Park. A backcountry permit is required for fires or overnight camping. See additional notes at the end of hike description regarding other considerations.

Directions

From Denver, take I-25 north to CO 66. Travel west through Longmont on CO 66 and then through Lyons. Take a left at the dead-end stoplight in Lyons and go west on CO 36 to Estes Park. Turn left off of CO 36 onto CO 7 before the first stoplight in Estes Park. Go south on CO 7, past Mary's Lake. The road curves sharply and travels to the Longs Peak trailhead turnoff. Turn right here and travel 1 mile to the Longs Peak trailhead.

GPS Trailhead Coordinates

UTM Zone (WGS84)   13T
Easting   0452659
Northing   4457866
Latitude   N 40.269928°
Longitude   W 105.556803°

A survey disk at Longs Peak placed by the U.S. Coast & Geodetic Survey.

face of Longs Peak. Head northwest as the trail skirts up Mount Lady Washington to Granite Pass.

Stay left and hike southwest for 1.7 miles to a boulder field. Within this boulder field is another pit toilet and several rock shelters that act as a windbreak for tents. The boulder field consists of car-sized boulders. Begin to scramble your way straight up toward the Keyhole. At the base of the boulder field, the top of Longs Peak, the Keyhole, and the expanse of the boulder field are visible.

Many people choose to backpack this far to make for a shorter climb the next day. All campers must obtain a backcountry wilderness use permit. Be warned that you are camping well above tree line, and the surface area is 100 percent rock.

The impressive view of the Longs Peak summit is highlighted here by a rock formation aptly dubbed the Keyhole. At the Keyhole is a small, stone shelter. The terrain becomes significantly more difficult beyond the Keyhole, so take a moment to evaluate the time, the weather, and your physical condition. There is no shame in turning back if the conditions aren't right; don't let pride get in the way of wisdom.

Cross through the Keyhole to the west side of the ridge and glance at an expansive view of Glacier Gorge. The trail is now marked by bull's eyes painted on the rocks. The remainder of the trail is extremely slick when wet and very exposed to the elements. A fall here could be fatal. Follow the exposed ledge for just over a quarter mile to a large couloir called the Trough. Ascend the Trough to the top of the west ridge.

Now the trail will traverse east across Longs Peak's south face using a ledge called the Narrows. This ledge is narrow—only one hiker wide—and exposed. Take your time and stay calm.

Beyond the Narrows lies the Homestretch. The Homestretch leads you northeast by a series of steep, slick, angled slabs. Be mindful of loose rock. Tread lightly, and watch for rock kicked loose by other hikers. In a short time, the summit of Longs Peak seems to just magically appear. This airy pinnacle is large and flat. The commanding panorama is well-deserved compensation for your sweat and tired legs. At 14,255 feet, plenty of photo opportunities exist.

After celebration of your lofty accomplishment, turn around and head back the way you came. The ascent will most likely be crowded, which can be a problem on the narrow ledges where hikers cannot pass each other.

Note: Hiking time and terrain warrant extra consideration when preparing for this outing. A headlamp is useful for an early start, which is essential for a successful completion of this hike. Many hikers begin as early as 2 a.m. Equip yourself with ample layers of clothing and extra food and water; this is a long one. As always, tell someone where you are going and when you expect to be back. An average of 60 search-and-rescue incidents occur per year on this peak alone. Crowds of hikers fill this trail every day. Be prepared for a lot of human contact. Snow is often found on this hike, especially through the Trough portion, at any time during the hiking season.

NEARBY ATTRACTIONS

Twin Sisters, Storm Pass Trail, and all Rocky Mountain National Park hikes. For more information: **estesparkcvb.com** or **nps.gov/romo**.

ROCKY MOUNTAIN NATIONAL PARK: STORM PASS TRAIL TO ESTES CONE 43

IN BRIEF

Estes Cone looks like an inactive volcano cone. In this book we will profile the trail from Longs Peak trailhead, even though two other access points lead to Estes Cone. This mostly shaded trail is a nice hike in the summer. It is also a good hike early or late in the season, when some other nearby hikes are thick with snow or impassable due to snow. Estes Cone is a Rocky Mountain National Park hike that can be accessed here without an entrance fee.

DESCRIPTION

Follow Longs Peak Trail from behind the little ranger's display and miniature museum at the parking lot. Please stop to sign in at the trail register right by the trailhead. Immediately ascend well-maintained man-made stairs. Since the trail is in Rocky Mountain National Park, hikers can expect a well-kept path throughout this hike, although the last half mile is rocky, steep, and hard to navigate.

The first half mile of trail is a steady, moderate grade that intersects with Storm Pass Trail. Take a right here onto Storm Pass Trail and follow the signs to Estes Cone.

The trail slowly gives way to loose rock and exposed tree roots. The grade varies as

KEY AT-A-GLANCE INFORMATION

LENGTH: 6.72 miles
CONFIGURATION: Out-and-back
DIFFICULTY: Difficult
SCENERY: Evergreen forest with spectacular mountain views at top
EXPOSURE: Shaded
TRAFFIC: Moderate
TRAIL SURFACE: Dirt with loose rock and tree roots
HIKING TIME: 3.5 hours
SEASON: May–October (open all year)
ACCESS: $20; open sunrise to sunset
MAPS: USGS Longs Peak
FACILITIES: Ranger station with ranger usually on duty, restrooms, campsites, and picnic facilities; museum, information on hikes and Rocky Mountain National Park
SPECIAL COMMENTS: Dogs are not allowed on any trail in Rocky Mountain National Park. A back-country permit is required for fires or overnight camping. This hike shares a trailhead with popular Longs Peak Trail. Many people start Longs Peak Trail at 4 or 5 a.m., finishing in early evening. Parking is limited, sometimes freeing up in the afternoon. However, an early start is recommended because lightning storms are common after 12 p.m.

Directions

From Denver, take I-25 north to CO 66. Travel west through Longmont on CO 66 and then through Lyons. Take a left at the dead-end stoplight in Lyons and go west on CO 36 to Estes Park. Turn left off of CO 36 onto CO 7 before the first stoplight in Estes Park. Go south on CO 7, past Mary's Lake. The road curves sharply and travels to the Longs Peak trailhead turnoff. Turn right here and travel 1 mile to the Longs Peak trailhead.

GPS Trailhead Coordinates

UTM Zone (WGS84) 13T
Easting 0452734
Northing 4457899
Latitude N 40.270230°
Longitude W 105.555923°

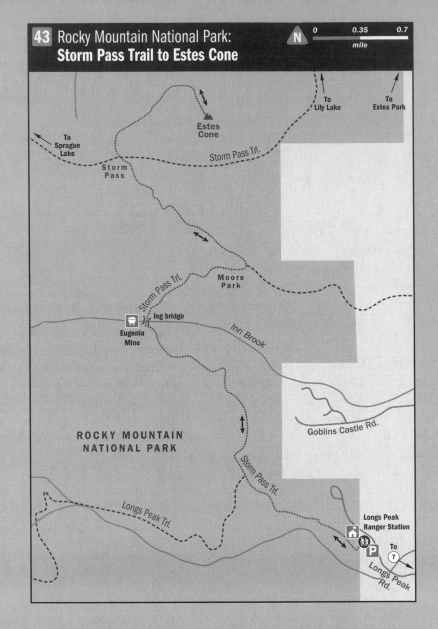

N

| 0 | 0.35 | 0.7 |
mile

To Lily Lake

To Estes Park

Estes Cone

To Sprague Lake

Storm Pass Trl.

Storm Pass

Moore Park

Storm Pass Trl.

log bridge

Eugenia Mine

Inn Brook

Goblins Castle Rd.

ROCKY MOUNTAIN NATIONAL PARK

Storm Pass Trl.

Longs Peak Trl.

Longs Peak Ranger Station

P

To 7

Longs Peak Rd.

10,500
10,000
9,500
9,000
8,500
8,000
7,500
7,000
6,500

FEET

0.5   1   1.5   2   2.5   3   3.36

MILES

Views and interesting rock outcrop along Storm Pass Trail to Estes Cone.

well, including some short descents and traverses below Pine Ridge. Cross Inn Brook using a log bridge and continue to the right of an abandoned log cabin site with a rusted boiler and tailings. This is all that remains of the Eugenia Mine.

The trail starts a descent that seems a little out of place, since our goal is to travel to a summit. Continue to drop down and cross a small meadow as the trail opens up to views of Twin Sisters and our destination, Estes Cone. The trail becomes sandy and smooth. Pass the Moore Park campsites, and at mile 2 reach a trail spur. Take a left, follow the signs to Estes Cone, and begin a sharp ascent toward Storm Pass. It is from this point that the trail makes up for lost time and gains most of its elevation.

To the left are spectacular views. The mountain to your far left is Mount Meeker. Longs Peak can be spotted poking above the ridge, with the peak's diamond facing the trail.

Lungs begin to tire as the elevation climbs and the trees become visibly shorter and stunted. At 2.5 miles, you reach the pass, marked by large rock cairns and signs. The Storm Pass Cutoff, to the right, is accessed at the Lily Lake trailhead. Follow the signs to Estes Cone Trail, bearing right up through rock cairns and the stunted evergreens that dot the hillside. Estes Cone is straight ahead and once out of the trees the trail begins to ascend the cone's southwest flank.

The trail is steep and rocky, with twisted and stunted wind-worn trees. A close look at some of these trees will show lightning damage.

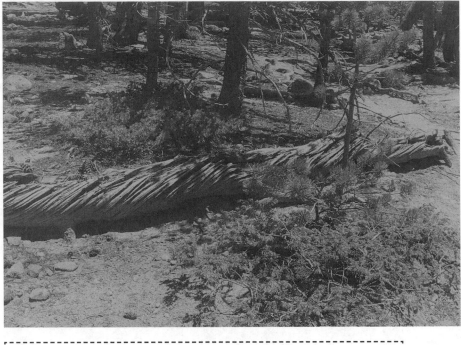

Look up and look down to truly appreciate the beauty of Storm Pass Trail to Estes Cone.

Continue to follow the cairns as you pick your way through a vertical rock garden for the last half mile. Eventually, reach a small flat area, then head up and right and scramble through rocks to the summit of Estes Cone. You are rewarded with magnificent views of Estes Park, Rocky Mountain National Park, Longs Peak, and Mount Meeker. But you should head down, back to the trailhead, before afternoon lightning storms return, as they do most of the summer.

NEARBY ATTRACTIONS

Twin Sisters, Longs Peak, and all Rocky Mountain National Park hikes. For more information: **estesparkcvb.com** or **nps.gov/romo**.

ROCKY MOUNTAIN NATIONAL PARK: TWIN SISTERS

44

IN BRIEF

The Twin Sisters sit at the easternmost edge of Rocky Mountain National Park and are accessed without entering the park. The trail winds through forest with some of the best panoramic views of Longs Peak. This is a great conditioning climb for those wanting to tackle considerable elevations.

DESCRIPTION

Start at Lily Lake Visitor Center. Get on the road right behind the visitor center and follow it away from the highway. At the official trailhead for Twin Sisters, take a left onto the trail. Start out on a small service road bordered on both sides by new evergreen tree growth. Immediately on the left is a small wooden bridge, Twin Sisters Trail information, and a trail marker.

Start a steady ascent on a trail comprised of loose rock and dirt. Enter a pine forest and then enter Forest Service land as the trees crowd and condense around the trail. Hikers ascend rather quickly and must scramble across some early rocks. The trail takes a deep right switchback and continues up the face of the mountain. The ascending path is aided in spots not only by switchbacks but also by man-made rock staircases. Continue to climb as scenery stays the

KEY AT-A-GLANCE INFORMATION

LENGTH: 8 miles

CONFIGURATION: Out-and-back

DIFFICULTY: Difficult

SCENERY: Views of Estes Park, Rocky Mountain National Park; optimal views of Longs Peak

EXPOSURE: Mostly shaded

TRAFFIC: Heavy

TRAIL SURFACE: Hard-packed dirt, some loose rocks

HIKING TIME: 4 hours

SEASON: May–October (open all year)

ACCESS: Free; open sunrise to sunset

MAPS: USGS Longs Peak

FACILITIES: Trailhead kiosk

SPECIAL COMMENTS: Dogs are not allowed on any trail in Rocky Mountain National Park. A backcountry permit is required for fires or overnight camping. The former Twin Sisters Trail, which began directly west of the summit in Tahosa Valley, has been abandoned by the National Park Service. Park at the Lily Lake Visitor Center and hike the extra 0.3 miles to avoid the nightmare parking along the road, right before the true trailhead.

Directions

From Denver, take I-25 north to CO 66. Travel west through Longmont on CO 66 and then through Lyons. Take a left at the dead-end stoplight in Lyons and go west on CO 36 to Estes Park. Turn left off of CO 36 onto CO 7 before the first stoplight in Estes Park. Go south on CO 7, past Mary's Lake. The road curves sharply and travels to Lily Lake Visitor Center on the left. Turn in here and park.

GPS Trailhead Coordinates

UTM Zone (WGS84) 13T

Easting 0454440

Northing 4461730

Latitude N 40.304838°

Longitude W 105.536132°

A nice peek and quick view of Longs Peak from a coveted spot on Twin Sisters Trail.

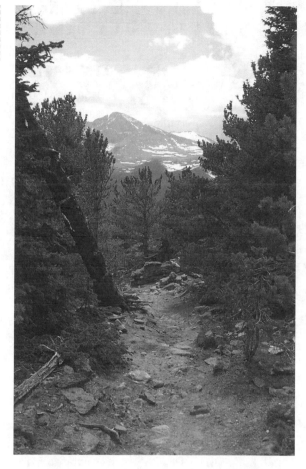

same. Cross a rockslide and enter into Rocky Mountain National Park. The trail becomes much steeper here, with a large staircase looming in the distance.

Turn and look to the right to capture the first amazing views of Longs Peak as it rises up over the Tahosa Valley. Pass through a second rockslide. Reach a small overlook and take in the view. Continue on as the trail starts a gradual descent, which is welcome since the previous steps have been straight uphill.

Pass a huge, five-story-tall boulder and then take artificially carved rock stairs up. The trail switches back again to the left and continues an uphill climb. Aspen trees have now begun to mix in with the tall, dense evergreens. Smaller switchbacks continue, and the trail is very rocky with exposed tree roots.

The trail continues its upward journey and then reaches an area with fewer trees, more shrubs, and small aspens. The trail is narrow and hard to navigate due to huge rocks in the path. Climb away from the hillside and leave the view of Longs Peak. Enter Forest Service land again and continue. After passing through timberline, keep going to the summit area and head past the communications tower. The true Twin Sisters summit is not directly accessible by trail but can be reached by a brief scramble heading east from the communications tower. Take in the views and head back the way you came.

NEARBY ATTRACTIONS

Lily Mountain, Lily Lake, Longs Peak, and all Rocky Mountain National Park hikes. For more information: **estesparkcvb.com** or **nps.gov/romo**.

45 ROUND MOUNTAIN: SUMMIT ADVENTURE TRAIL

KEY AT-A-GLANCE INFORMATION

LENGTH: 9.84 miles

CONFIGURATION: Out-and-back

DIFFICULTY: Difficult

SCENERY: Subalpine, dense pine trees, large boulders, views of Big Thompson Canyon

EXPOSURE: Shaded, cool; exposed, hot. (Be prepared to be hot in spring/summer and cold in fall/winter)

TRAFFIC: Mild

TRAIL SURFACE: Loose dirt and rock, exposed tree roots

HIKING TIME: 6 hours

SEASON: May–October

ACCESS: Free; open sunrise to sunset

MAPS: USGS Drake; Foothills Nature Trail maps at trailhead

FACILITIES: Restroom, trailhead register

SPECIAL COMMENTS: Foothills Interpretive Nature Trail and Summit Adventure Trail both originate from Round Mountain trailhead. The main Round Mountain hike is the Summit Adventure Trail, featured here. The Foothills Nature Trail is an interpretive, 1-mile nature hike. A significant portion of the trail lies directly above CO 34, so expect traffic noise from the canyon.

IN BRIEF

Round Mountain is a difficult hike to the summit of Sheep Mountain above the Big Thompson River and Canyon. The trail is a steady uphill grade with a forgiving and welcome descent after the summit. It is easy to navigate, with mile markers and informational signs full of trail trivia.

DESCRIPTION

This challenging hike begins on the Foothills Nature Trail, an interpretive trail that is part of the Round Mountain National Recreation Trail. From the parking area, walk past the restroom, sign in at the hiking register, and continue up a wide gravel road. Do not be deceived by the undemanding beginning; the first 0.25 miles overlaps with the easy interpretive trail, but the majority of this hike takes hikers up the side of the Big Thompson Canyon, over the Continental Divide, and to the top of Sheep Mountain. The Summit Adventure Trail also serves as an interpretive trail, with several information plaques. When I hiked with my friends Sarah and Shannon, we found that the plaques were spaced just right, giving us time to stop and catch our breath if we needed to, while learning about the natural history of the area.

GPS Trailhead Coordinates

UTM Zone (WGS84) 13T

Easting 0475840

Northing 4474232

Latitude N 40.418363°

Longitude W 105.284783°

Directions

From Denver, take I-25 north to CO 34 west through Loveland. Travel 4 miles on CO 34 west of the Dam Store in the Big Thompson Canyon. Turn left into the small dirt parking lot across the highway from the entrance of Vistenz-Smith Park. You will pass the Loveland Power Plant on the right.

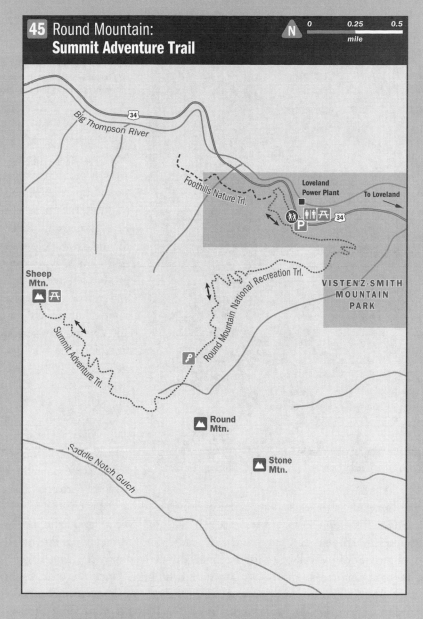

45 Round Mountain:
Summit Adventure Trail

N   0   0.25   0.5
mile

Big Thompson River
34

Foothills Nature Trl.

Loveland
Power Plant

To Loveland

84

P

Sheep
Mtn.

VISTENZ-SMITH
MOUNTAIN
PARK

Round Mountain National Recreation Trl.

Summit Adventure Trl.

Round
Mtn.

Saddle Notch Gulch

Stone
Mtn.

8,500

8,000

7,500

7,000

6,500

6,000

FEET 5,500

5,000

4,500

1   2   3   4   4.92

MILES

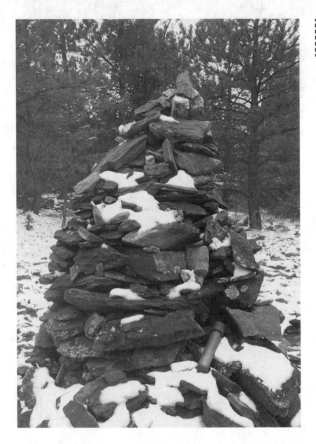

A six-foot-high man-made rock formation marks the summit.

The two trails split at a well-marked fork. Take a left onto the Summit Trail and begin an immediate climb on a dirt-and-rock trail that runs parallel to the Big Thompson River and the highway below. As the trail climbs, it narrows and produces steep drop-offs and exposed tree roots. Continue climbing and climbing and climbing. Instead of cutting directly across the ridge of the canyon, the trail begins a series of unforgiving switchbacks that route hikers up the mountainside. This steep incline, in addition to being a lung buster, is heavily eroded in places. Natural erosion has even carved magnificent rock sculptures out of boulders along the trail.

The first mile takes hikers through national forest land, and the trail is extremely narrow, rocky, and shaded. Already, the trail meanders through a variety of vegetation: yuccas, Spanish bayonets or small soapweed, fringed sagebrush, ponderosa pine trees, and Rocky Mountain junipers. Once the trail reaches the canyon top, it breaks onto exposed hillsides that can be quite sunbathed in the summer. Continuing on the second mile of the climb are more drop-offs and new views of the northeastern plains. It is necessary to have some nontechnical bouldering skills, since you must maneuver through chasms between towering rock formations. These rock formations jettison out of the mountain like mythical guardians of the trail.

Once through the passage, the trail opens up to aspen trees and a small spring that gurgles out of the mountainside. The trail descends a bit after the third mile, and views of Round Mountain's top are prevalent for the last mile or so. A small aspen forest lines the path, and then the trail ascends again into a less exposed forest of Douglas fir and various pines.

Although Round Mountain is the hike's namesake, this is not the final destination. The Summit Adventure Trail takes hikers to the top of Sheep Mountain. The

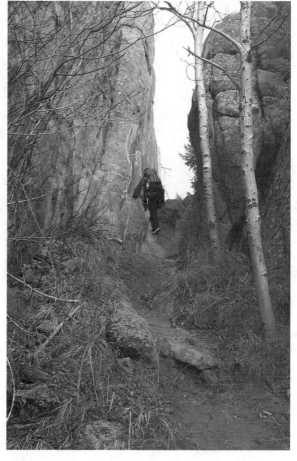

Steep inclines challenge hikers.

hike is also referred to as Dome Mountain, but locals have never wavered from the Round Mountain title.

The summit of the trail, approximately 8,500 feet above sea level (and 2,250-2,750 feet from where you began) is sheltered by a halo of trees. Take a deep, long breath, and be sure to sign the trail log at the summit. The summit is marked by a six-foot-high, man-made stack of rocks. There is a nice picnic area to relax and rest.

Round Mountain is a hike of extremes, so the strain of the ascent is remedied by the sloping descent. After a respite at the summit, head downhill and sign out at the hike register.

NEARBY ATTRACTIONS

Foothills Nature Trail, part of the Round Mountain National Recreation Trail, is an easy alternative if you're short on time.

SOUTH OF DENVER
(INCLUDING COLORADO SPRINGS)

46 BEAR CREEK CAÑON PARK: PALMER RED ROCK LOOP

KEY AT-A-GLANCE INFORMATION

LENGTH: 5.72 miles

CONFIGURATION: Loop

DIFFICULTY: Difficult

SCENERY: Foothills, evergreen forest, views of Colorado Springs and plains

EXPOSURE: Mostly shaded except for full exposure in the first mile

TRAFFIC: Moderate

TRAIL SURFACE: Hard-packed dirt

HIKING TIME: 3 hours

SEASON: All year

ACCESS: Free; open sunrise to sunset

MAPS: USGS Manitou Springs

FACILITIES: None

SPECIAL COMMENTS: Trail signs seem to be missing, and limited information—including an information board, faded map, and info on how the trailhead, called Section 16, got its name—at trailhead. Land in the West is based on the township and range system of dividing parcels of land, which includes sections. A section is 1 square mile, and in the 1800s, proceeds from leases to sections numbered 16 and 36 were designated for schools. El Paso County Parks leases section 16 and uses it as Bear Creek Cañon Park. An independent group has named this trail Ring the Peak Trail.

IN BRIEF

Many of the hikes in Colorado Springs are great but also short and easy. At 6 miles and with a difficult rating, the Palmer Red Rock Loop is a break from the norm. The trail takes hikers on a loop in the foothills on the western edge of Colorado Springs. The first half of the loop ascends and the second half descends.

DESCRIPTION

Start at the Section 16 trailhead and take the Palmer Red Rock Loop. The singletrack trail goes through miniature oak trees that are a little bigger than the area's scrub oak, but definitely not full trees. The path switchbacks up the hillside and provides great views of downtown Colorado Springs. Follow the trail north. As you climb, you'll see bigger views, including a small portion of Bear Creek Cañon Park. Here, the oaks start giving way to yuccas. Social trails abound in the first stretch of this hike, but the main trail is always obvious. The trail turns to red dirt, descends, and levels out for awhile with views toward Garden of the Gods.

About 0.75 miles into the hike, you come to an intersection with the Intenman Nature Trail. Continue straight. (A right turn here takes hikers to the east edge of Manitou

GPS Trailhead Coordinates

UTM Zone (WGS84) 13S

Easting 0509520

Northing 4296910

Latitude N 38.820921°

Longitude W 104.890335°

Directions

From Denver, take I-25 south to Colorado Springs. Take exit 141, which is CO 24, and go left. Take a left on 26th Street and drive up into the foothills a little bit. At the stop sign, turn right on Gold Camp Road and go a mile to the trailhead and parking area on the right. If that parking lot is full, continue another 100 yards, and a parking area is on the left.

Intenman Nature Trl.

Ring the Peak Trl.

Palmer Red Rock Loop

Gold Camp Rd.

Bear Creek Rd.

To
Colorado
Springs

P

Gold Camp Rd.

Palmer Red Rock Trl.

Hunter Run

Ring the Peak Trl.

High Drive

Bear Creek

**BEAR CREEK
CAÑON PARK**

Bear Creek

High Drive

8,500

8,000

7,500

7,000

6,500

6,000

5,500

5,000

4,500

FEET

1   2   3   4   5   5.72

MILES

Views of the plains and of Colorado Springs can be seen from the trail in Bear Creek Cañon Park.

Springs, while a left turn leads to the Forest Overlook.) A map is posted at this intersection. The trail continues on Palmer Red Rock Trail and is also marked as Ring the Peak Trail. In 300 yards, you'll see an alternate right turn to the Intenman Trail; keep going straight.

While steep, the trail offers shade as you enter the evergreen trees. Come to a T; take a left. After eight switchbacks and a lot of steep climbing, come to a well-defined line where the trees thin. A left here goes to a scenic overlook, but the main trail switchbacks to the right and continues climbing. When you come to the top of the ridge, you'll be treated to a scenic view of tree-covered foothills and a glimpse of The Broadmoor, a historic, landmark hotel. A left here goes to several scenic overlooks; a right will keep you on the main trail. This is a noticeable change of direction heading west, traversing the mountainside. Continue to follow the Ring the Peak signs. As the trail starts to descend, you cross open, yucca-covered areas with wide sun exposure.

As the trail curves to the left, starting to loop back toward the trailhead, you enter an obvious change in ecological zones. A notably cool, dense spruce forest is located right after the yuccas. The steep hillside doesn't allow for much sun here except the morning eastern sun. To the left you see Colorado Springs across the plains.

The trail travels downward gradually and steadily, traversing the surrounding mountains. You are actually doing a big U-turn, always turning to the left,

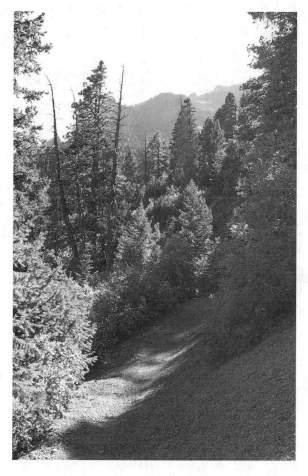

A small section of trail along
Palmer Red Rock Loop.

eventually pointing east on the other side of the valley. Continue going east in a straight line for 0.75 miles, and the trail will start to wind around again. Continue a very gradual descent and drop down into Bear Creek Cañon. At the trail intersection in Bear Creek Cañon, take a left and continue downhill on Ring the Peak Trail. Another 200 yards down the trail, the trail forks. Go right and stay on the main trail.

When you reach a dirt road, High Drive, turn left and walk down the single-lane, dirt road. The last mile of this hike is on the road, used mostly by bikes and closed to cars. Proceed through the gate, where the road is now paved, and come to a stop sign. Turn left onto Gold Camp Road and go uphill, noting the rock formations above and to the left. Another few minutes' walk will take you back to the car.

47 BLODGETT PEAK OPEN SPACE: WATER TANK TRAIL

KEY AT-A-GLANCE INFORMATION

LENGTH: 2 miles

CONFIGURATION: Out-and-back

DIFFICULTY: Easy

SCENERY: Pine trees, thick scrub oak, cliff views

EXPOSURE: No shade

TRAFFIC: Moderate

TRAIL SURFACE: Wide, dirt utility road

HIKING TIME: 50 minutes

SEASON: All year

ACCESS: Free; open sunrise to sunset

MAPS: USGS Cascade

FACILITIES: Portable toilet

SPECIAL COMMENTS: Dogs must be leashed. A city ordinance stresses the importance of dog refuse removal. No model rocket launches.

IN BRIEF

Once part of the Blodgett Ranch, the Blodgett Peak Open Space area offers 167 acres of open space, trails, and wildlife habitat. The Water Tank Trail takes hikers along an old utility road and past unique geological rock features. Most of the land and rock formations are visible from numerous points around Colorado Springs. A pair of peregrine falcons was released at Eagle Peak, located north of Blodgett Peak.

DESCRIPTION

The utility road begins at the eastern boundary between two drainage basins. Leave the parking lot and pass the gate and the portable toilet. The trail begins to wind through scrub oak until it reaches the water tank. The property's lowest elevation is 7,054 feet, and the elevation rises sharply at the water tank on its western boundary at 8,184 feet at the end of this trail.

The trail curves to the left; follow it around the hillside. The path is a wide, dirt utility road that stays consistent and smooth through the entire hike. At the fork, stay right on the main trail. A smaller jogging trail has been cut into the grass along the utility road.

GPS Trailhead Coordinates

UTM Zone (WGS84) 13S

Easting 0509880

Northing 4310630

Latitude N 38.944555°

Longitude W 104.885990°

Directions

From Denver, take I-25 south to Colorado Springs. Take exit 149 and turn right, going west on Woodmen Road. At the intersection of Woodmen Road and Rockrimmon Road, turn right. Travel 5 miles through residential area until you reach the trailhead on the right, at 3898 West Woodmen Road.

47 Blodgett Peak Open Space:
Water Tank Trail

0   0.05   0.1
mile

N

To Colorado Springs and 25

Blodgett Dr.

Dry Creek

Blodgett Dr.

Angelstone Ct.

W. Woodmen Rd.

To Colorado Springs and 25

Water Tank Trl.

Water Tank Trl.

Water Tank

Water Tank Trl.

Dry Creek

BLODGETT PEAK OPEN SPACE

PIKE NATIONAL FOREST

8,500
8,000
7,500
7,000
6,500
6,000
5,500
5,000
4,500

FEET

0.25   0.5   0.75   1

MILES

View of Colorado Springs from Water Tank Trail.

Much of the property is dominated by gambrel oaks and ponderosa pines. On the north-facing slopes, Douglas fir is prevalent because of cooler temperatures and greater moisture available. As the trail continues to ascend, the trees become dense.

The trail continues to ascend and curves gently up the hillside. Views to the west, directly in front of hikers, are the nesting cliffs of Blodgett Peak and Eagle Peak. You don't have to look close to see the falcons playing above. Behind you, to the east, are views of Colorado Springs.

At the water tank, turn around and head back the way you came. Future trails are planned in this new open space that will travel beyond the water tower and connect to Pike National Forest and other trails. Pike National Forest borders Blodgett Peak Open Space on three sides.

NEARBY ATTRACTIONS

Other Colorado Springs area hikes, including the Foothills Trail and the Woodmen Trail, plus the nearby Oak Valley Ranch Park: **springsgov.com/parks**.

CASTLEWOOD CANYON STATE PARK: INNER CANYON LOOP 48

IN BRIEF

Castlewood Canyon is the northernmost portion of the Black Forest. Largely surrounded by grassland, the canyon is home to dam ruins. The Inner Canyon Loop takes hikers through a lush corridor where ponderosa pines thrive along Cherry Creek as it flows to Denver. Castlewood Canyon State Park has 12 miles of hiking trails, including the handicap-accessible Canyon View Nature Trail.

DESCRIPTION

Leave the parking area and go to the Lake Gulch trailhead. Pass by the restrooms, picnic area, and the playground. Concrete at the beginning, the wide path's surface then turns into dirt and loose rocks. On the left is the turnoff for the Pikes Peak Amphitheater.

The trail begins to gradually descend, and views to the left open up to the valley below.

Ranches and residential areas become visible. The trail now skirts over large boulders but is still easy to navigate. Here, the path is narrow, and foliage hugs the sides. Start to wind downward. The trail is cut into the hillside here: If you reach your right hand out, you can touch the hillside; on your left, the hill drops down.

KEY AT-A-GLANCE INFORMATION

LENGTH: 1.8 miles
CONFIGURATION: Loop
DIFFICULTY: Easy
SCENERY: Ponderosa pine, piñon pine, scrub oak, high plains, canyon overlooks, distant view of the mountains
EXPOSURE: Little shade
TRAFFIC: Moderate
TRAIL SURFACE: Hard-packed dirt, smooth
HIKING TIME: 1 hour
SEASON: All year
ACCESS: $6 state park fee; only open during daytime hours; park opens at 8 a.m. and closing time varies by season
MAPS: USGS Russellville Gulch, South Castle Rock
FACILITIES: Visitor center, restroom, playground, covered picnic area, amphitheater
SPECIAL COMMENTS: Dogs must be on a leash that cannot exceed six feet in length. Most areas in the park are handicap accessible. No horses.

Directions

From Denver, take I-25 south to Castle Rock, turn east on CO 86, going right, and go 6 miles to Franktown. Turn right, going south on CO 83 (South Parker Road), and go 5 miles south to the park entrance on the right. Pay at the visitor center drive-through window and proceed to the east facilities, Canyon Point.

GPS Trailhead Coordinates

UTM Zone (WGS84) 13S
Easting 0522010
Northing 4353570
Latitude N 39.331269°
Longitude W 104.744624'

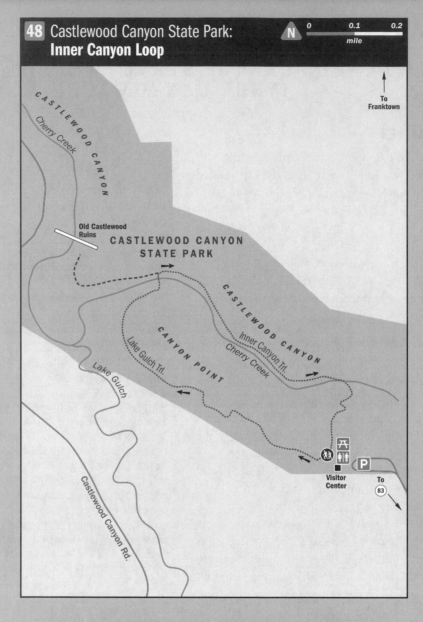

N

0   0.1   0.2
mile

To
Franktown

C A S T L E W O O D C A N Y O N

Cherry Creek

Old Castlewood
Ruins

**CASTLEWOOD CANYON
STATE PARK**

C A S T L E W O O D C A N Y O N

Inner Canyon Trl.
Cherry Creek

Lake Gulch Trl.

C A N Y O N P O I N T

Lake Gulch

Castlewood Canyon Rd.

Visitor
Center

P

To
83

8,500
8,000
7,500
7,000
6,500
6,000
5,500
5,000
4,500

FEET

0.5   1   1.5   1.8

MILES

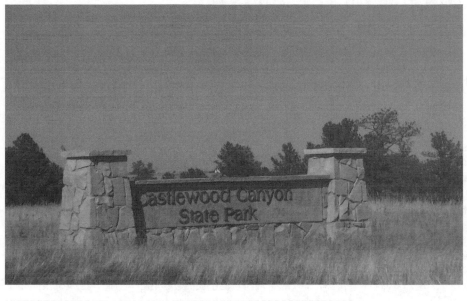

A sign that greets visitors at the turnoff to Castlewood Canyon State Park.

Erosion-control devices such as hand-laid logs can be found throughout the descent. The trail begins to curve to the right. To the left is a small gully and canyon walls. Forest still dominates the right.

Next, the trail narrows, with grass on both sides. Cherry Creek fills the gully; cross the stream via a wooden footbridge. Climb stairs and come to the intersection of Lake Gulch Trail, Inner Canyon Trail, and Dam Ruins. Continue straight up the hill on Inner Canyon Trail, which then begins to descend. As you climb through rocks, you'll hear the sound of trickling from Cherry Creek. The trail levels a little, crosses a small wooden bridge, then another. Stay on the designated trail. No scrambling is required on the large boulders. Just walk over or through them.

Climb another set of man-made stairs and begin a set of switchbacks. Pass a dead tree and cross another bridge. Walk over the dry streambed, cross another bridge, and start another ascent through high scrub oak. Canyon ledges and boulders line the dirt trail.

Come to a little erosion area near the creek that looks like theater seating and pass behind it. Cross two more bridges over Cherry Creek. On the other side of the creek, the trail ascends via gentle switchbacks. Stairs are located in steeper places. Reach an actual staircase and at the top, pass an Inner Canyon trailhead sign and go right. The trail is now concrete and heads directly back to the car.

NEARBY ATTRACTIONS

Try the other Castlewood Canyon State Park hikes. The longest trail is the Rimrock Loop at 2.14 miles: **parks.state.co.us**.

49   COLORADO TRAIL: LITTLE SCRAGGY TRAIL

KEY AT-A-GLANCE INFORMATION

LENGTH: 11.48 miles

CONFIGURATION: Out-and-back

DIFFICULTY: Moderate

SCENERY: Forested, rock formations, distant views of mountains

EXPOSURE: Mostly shaded

TRAFFIC: Moderate

TRAIL SURFACE: Extremely smooth and hard-packed dirt

HIKING TIME: 5 hours

SEASON: All year

ACCESS: $4; open sunrise to sunset

MAPS: USGS Green Mountain

FACILITIES: Restroom, information kiosk

SPECIAL COMMENTS: Dogs must be leashed. This is a short section of the Colorado Trail, which runs more than 400 miles from Denver to Durango. Hikers may encounter large mountain-bike crowds as well as backpackers doing long trips.

IN BRIEF

The Little Scraggy Trail features 11.48 miles of Colorado's landmark 475-mile-long Colorado Trail and part of Colorado Trail Segment 3. This winding, wooded trail has great views and rock formations. Hikers encounter a naturally smooth trail surface that is easy to navigate. This moderate hike will not leave you the least bit scraggy.

DESCRIPTION

From the parking lot, cross over toward the restroom. Turn left on the singletrack trail near the information kiosk. Start hiking as the trail winds through a lush pine forest. Eventually come to Forest Service Road 550 and cross straight over the road as the trail continues its twists and turns. The trail is memorable for its smooth path lined with ponderosa pines and a smattering of lodgepole pines. It remains relatively level as it travels through the Buffalo Creek Area. The namesake Little Scraggy Peak is always to the left, although it is never quite visible.

Pass an overlook with striking rock formations where you can see for miles in all directions. On a clear day, the southern views may open up to Pikes Peak. Pass the intersection with Shinglemill Trail. Bear left,

GPS Trailhead Coordinates

UTM Zone (WGS84) 13S

Easting   0477870

Northing 4354860

Latitude   N 39.342890°

Longitude W 105.256811°

Directions

From Denver, take C 470 south to US 285 west. Travel 21 miles to Pine Junction, and turn left on CO 126. Go south for 13 miles until you see a sign for the Colorado Trail on the right side of CO 126 at FS 550. Take a quick right into the parking lot at the trailhead.

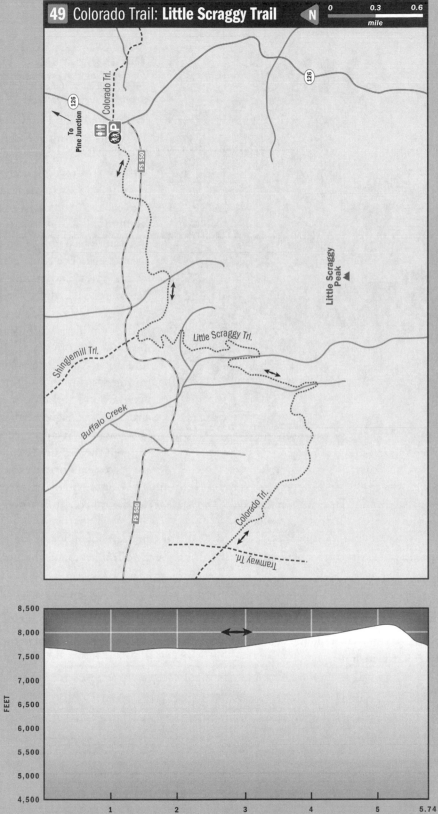

N

0   0.3   0.6
mile

126

To
Pine Junction

Colorado Trl.

P

FS 550

Little Scraggy
Peak

Little Scraggy Trl.

Shinglemill Trl.

Buffalo Creek

FS 550

Colorado Trl.

Tramway Trl.

FEET

8,500

8,000

7,500

7,000

6,500

6,000

5,500

5,000

4,500

1   2   3   4   5   5.74

MILES

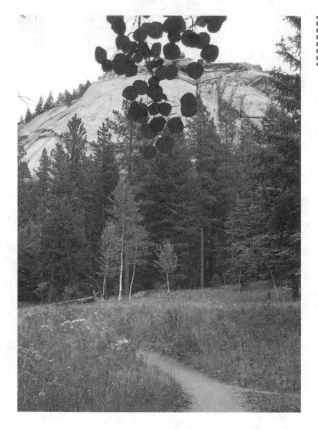

Little Scraggy Trail rock outcrops typical of those seen throughout most of the hike.

go downhill, and stay on the main Colorado Trail. This is a gradual hill, and halfway down, you'll access wide-open views. At the bottom of the descent, you'll find aspen groves and a little lush gully. Cross a tiny creek. The trail veers to the right and parallels the creek for a while. After the lush section, emerge into a familiar wildflower meadow with pine trees. Be sure to stay on the main trail here as it continues to wind around and loop in a circle to the right. Other, lesser-used trails cut through the meadow.

Continue on this trail, through the forest, and up through meadows. Eventually, you'll parallel another creek and then intersect with Tramway Trail, where we end our hike. Turn around here and go back the way you came.

You may continue on the Colorado Trail for hundreds of miles or travel one way the entire 13.5-mile length to the Rolling Creek Trailhead and the Lost Creek Wilderness Area.

NEARBY ATTRACTIONS

Colorado Trail: **coloradotrail.org**. Other Pike National Forest trails: **fs.fed.us/r2/psicc/recreation/trails**.

DOUGLAS COUNTY OPEN SPACE: GLENDALE FARM TRAIL

50

IN BRIEF

Glendale Farm Trail sits in a region called Happy Canyon. So think of this as a happy hike. It's a great first-time hike for kids or novices because of the short length and easy navigation. No shade means that the midsummer heat can be unbearable. Douglas County Open Space does an amazing job on these new trails. They are usually complete with benches and picnic tables placed along the way. Color information and history brochures are available at the trailhead.

DESCRIPTION

From the end of the parking lot, go straight through the fence, hike 50 feet, and take a right turn. Travel counterclockwise on the loop and begin hiking among scrub oak, prairie grasses, and sagebrush. Glendale Farm consists of short-grass prairie and shrubs. Pronghorn antelope, coyotes, cottontail rabbits, prairie dogs, mule deer, black bears, red foxes, and rattlesnakes all make this land their home.

The loop winds uphill a little at first. Once hikers arrive at the back corner, the easternmost part of the trail, the grade levels out and gets easier as the trail continues north. From here, you'll enjoy views of Glendale Farm's 160 acres and distant panoramas of the

KEY AT-A-GLANCE INFORMATION

LENGTH: 1.5 miles
CONFIGURATION: Loop
DIFFICULTY: Easy
SCENERY: Foothills and rolling plains
EXPOSURE: No shade
TRAFFIC: Moderate
TRAIL SURFACE: Hard-packed dirt, some loose rocks
HIKING TIME: 40 minutes
SEASON: All year
ACCESS: Free; open sunrise to sunset
MAPS: USGS Castle Rock North
FACILITIES: Portable restrooms, picnic facilities, horse-hitching rails, emergency phones
SPECIAL COMMENTS: A fenced, five-acre off-leash dog park is located southwest of the main trailhead and is perfect for letting the dog run before hiking the trail. Once on the trail, dogs must be leashed. Rattlesnakes live in this area. Climbing on the rocks is not allowed.

Directions ————————➤

From Denver, take I-25 south to the Surrey Ridge exit (number 190). Travel east under the highway, take a quick left, and you'll see the parking lot from there.

GPS Trailhead Coordinates

UTM Zone (WGS84) 13S
Easting 0511220
Northing 4371097
Latitude N 39.489407°
Longitude W 104.869523°

GLENDALE FARM
OPEN SPACE

Clydesdale Rd.

To
Denver

25

25

Oak Ln.

Glendale Farm Trl.

The easy loop at Glendale Farm Open Space offers no shade.

mountains. Although the farm buildings no longer stand, remnants on this trail, such as the barnyard and orchard, remind hikers of the dedicated spirit of early pioneers. One such pioneer was so happy that he could always be heard singing as he rode over these hills. His happiness echoed through the valley and gave this region its name, Happy Canyon.

Continue along the trail. Approaching a barbed-wire fence, the trail curves to the left, going west, and then meets a fork. The right fork goes to a scenic overlook that is not recommended because of the proximity of I-25, so take a left, wind downhill, and end up back at the trailhead.

NEARBY ATTRACTIONS

Other Douglas County Open Space trails: **douglas.co.us.**

51 DOUGLAS COUNTY OPEN SPACE: GREENLAND TRAIL

KEY AT-A-GLANCE INFORMATION

LENGTH: 8.5 miles
CONFIGURATION: Loop
DIFFICULTY: Easy
SCENERY: Mountain views, plains, Pikes Peak
EXPOSURE: No shade
TRAFFIC: Light
TRAIL SURFACE: Smooth, hard-packed dirt
HIKING TIME: 3 hours
SEASON: All year
ACCESS: Free; open sunrise to sunset
MAPS: USGS Greenland, Larkspur
FACILITIES: Portable restrooms, picnic shelter, covered horse-hitch rails, water spigot, emergency telephone
SPECIAL COMMENTS: Dogs must be leashed. Take plenty of water and know your limitations. Water is available at the trailhead. The land outside the fences is privately owned. An accessible group picnic shelter, patterned after Greenland's old mercantile building, seats up to 48 people. Benches, hitch rails, and picnic tables can be found along the trail.

IN BRIEF

The Greenland Trail, within roughly 3,000 acres of Greenland Open Space, winds through rolling grasslands, a pond, scrub oaks, and pine forests. This scenic hike is right off of I-25 and offers easy access.

DESCRIPTION

Leave the parking area and proceed past the picnic shelter, heading south. The trail is wide, smooth-packed dirt. After the trail travels alongside the Old Territorial Trail, it will intersect with the Kipps Loop portion of the Greenland Trail. Take a left turn at this intersection and begin to travel clockwise around the loop. All turns along the trail are well marked.

The trail ascends and the trail surface softens for the next mile. As you climb, the sights and sounds of I-25 begin to disappear behind the ridge to the left. Take a short respite under the trees here, as they provide rare shade along the trail. Pass a small burn area from 2002, along with a picnic table and a horse-hitching rail.

The trail descends for a short time and then begins another gradual uphill climb. As it gets close to the low scrub oaks, you soon reach the highest point in the path. Start a small descent and pass another group of trees, a picnic table, and a hitching rail.

GPS Trailhead Coordinates

UTM Zone (WGS84) 13S
Easting 0512710
Northing 4336590
Latitude N 39.178450°
Longitude W 104.852849°

Directions

From Denver, take I-25 south (south of Larkspur and north of Palmer Lake) to the Greenland exit, number 167. Take a right, going west on CR 74. Travel 0.75 miles, and continue straight into the parking lot.

N

0   0.4   0.8
mile

18

E. Greenland Rd.

Greenland
Schoolhouse

25

P

E. Greenland Rd.

Eagle Mtn.

S. Spruce Mtn. Rd.

18

Greenland Trl.

Old Territorial
Trl.

Spruce
Mtn.

Greenland Trl.

Kips Loop

25

18

Bald Mtn.

GREENLAND
OPEN SPACE

To
Monument

25

County Line Rd.

8,500

8,000

7,500

7,000

6,500

6,000

5,500

5,000

4,500

FEET

2   4   6   8   8.5

MILES

Why not take a short respite on this bench along the flat and fairly easy Greenland Trail?

A 19th-century grave marker also marks the farthest point in the loop. This large spherical monument, which is fenced among the trees and very elaborate, pays tribute to Edward Kipps, an area pioneer.

Greenland was once a bustling village with two general stores, a post office, a school, and a saloon. In 1871, the Denver & Rio Grande Railroad extended to this site, and the two railroad stations shipped out everything from livestock to pottery. The ranching industry continued after the town's decline in the 1930s.

The next few miles descend and the trail is in plain sight as hikers cross the prairie. At the bottom of the hill, with the railroad tracks straight ahead, take a right turn as the trail forks. Continue straight on the easy road for a mile to the intersection with Old Territorial Road. Bear right and go uphill, staying on the Greenland Trail and getting off the road. Wind up and over a small hill, past a pond, and continue back in the direction of the trailhead.

NEARBY ATTRACTIONS

Spruce Meadows Trail is nearby, along with other Douglas County Open Space hikes: **douglas.co.us**.

FLORISSANT FOSSIL BEDS: PETRIFIED FOREST LOOP 52

IN BRIEF

Prehistoric Colorado is preserved in this unique national monument. Petrified red-wood tree stumps, insect fossils, plant fossils, and more reveal one of the most diverse fossil deposits discovered in the West. Eight diverse trails weave in and out of the remains and offer different vantage points of the Florissant Fossil Beds history. The Petrified Forest Loop is a great starter trail and passes many of the more popular sites, such as the famed Big Stump and the Scudder excavation pit.

DESCRIPTION

Start this hike by viewing the 14-minute orientation film, geologic exhibits, and fossil displays in the visitor center. The bookstore and the restrooms are also located here. Leave the visitor center and go behind the building where the hike begins. Pass an outdoor exhibit area and amphitheater, where you can see petrified redwood tree stumps and associated exhibits. In the summer, rangers give hourly talks here.

From the outdoor exhibit area, you have access to two self-guided trails—Walk Thru Time/Ponderosa Loop Trail and Petrified Forest Loop. Access the paved path and take a right turn onto the gravel path, partially shaded by small ponderosa tree stands. Continue on the

KEY AT-A-GLANCE INFORMATION

LENGTH: 1.1 miles
CONFIGURATION: Loop
DIFFICULTY: Easy
SCENERY: Meadow; petrified wood, fossils, and rocks
EXPOSURE: Sunny
TRAFFIC: Moderate
TRAIL SURFACE: Dirt
HIKING TIME: 30 minutes
SEASON: All year
ACCESS: $3 (good for 7 days) per person charge; ages 16 and younger free
MAPS: USGS Lake George
FACILITIES: Restrooms, visitor center, picnic area, bookstore
SPECIAL COMMENTS: Dogs and bikes are prohibited. Collecting any petrified artifacts is prohibited.

Directions

From Denver, take I-25 south to US 24, travel 35 miles to the town of Florissant, and then follow signs 2 miles south to the visitor center on Teller County 1.

GPS Trailhead Coordinates

UTM Zone (WGS84) 13T
Easting   0475350
Northing 4307031
Latitude N 38.911832°
Longitude W 105.284316°

Hornbek Homestead—complete with a bunkhouse, carriage shed, barn, and root cellar—is in view throughout your visit to the Florissant Fossil Beds.

Petrified Forest Loop, heading north toward the meadow. The main trail is a loop that begins here and passes self-guided tour posts and information signs.

The trail continues right and ascends; pass a bench overlooking a historic excavation site. Pass another bench before the trail turns right (east) and heads across the meadow. To the north are the outbuildings of the Hornbek Homestead. The last portion of the trail is set up as a time line, with every few inches of the trail representing the passage of a million years.

This 1.1-mile trail passes massive petrified redwood stumps, a historic excavation site, and a geological time line exhibit. This gravel trail is relatively flat and is mostly out in the open—a consideration during the hot, summer months. The trail ends back at the visitor center.

All of the ancient trees, now petrified artifacts, were preserved by volcanic mudflows and volcanic ash that occurred millions of years ago. Almost 100 stumps of giant sequoia redwood trees stand in the Florissant Fossil Beds, but most remain buried to preserve them. One of the largest is 13 feet in diameter and 42 feet around. When this tree was alive, in a very different, humid climate, this redwood may have stood 300 feet high and was at least 700 years old.

Use the Petrified Forest Loop as a jumping-off point for the other trails in the area. The Petrified Forest Loop is the longest of the two self-guided trails (brochures are available at the desk). The Walk Thru Time/Ponderosa Loop is 0.5 miles, and it is completely handicap accessible.

The massive petrified stump—affectionately called "Big Stump"—measures 38 feet in circumference.

The Hornbek Wildlife Loop is 4 miles and follows the meadow to the Hornbek Homestead and crosses land once covered by Lake Florissant. The return route overlooks the ancient lake bed and the mountain ranges beyond.

The Sawmill Trail is a 2.2-mile loop and offers varied terrain: forests of pine, spruce, and fir; meadows frequented by elk; ridgetops with a view of Pikes Peak; and shaded streams. The Hans Loop is an extension of the Sawmill. Part of the trail follows a gentle ridge that provides vistas of Pikes Peak and then drops into a drainage basin that passes the remnants of a rustic cabin.

The Boulder Creek Trail is a 3.2-mile loop that begins and ends in the ponderosa pine forest. A portion of the trail follows through wet meadows and past a formation of giant eroded granite boulders.

The 2.2-mile one-way Twin Rock Trail follows riparian (stream) habitat. And the 2.2-mile Shooting Star Trail follows an old roadbed. It was named after the nearby Shootin' Star Ranch.

NEARBY ATTRACTIONS

A visit to Cripple Creek is always fun: **cripple-creek.co.us.**

GARDEN OF THE GODS: PERKINS CENTRAL GARDEN TRAIL 53

IN BRIEF

Garden of the Gods is a must-see, ranking up there with Pikes Peak and the U.S. Air Force Academy, for any visitor to Colorado Springs. Garden of the Gods features 19 significant rock formations, and Perkins Central Garden Trail passes around more than half of them. This easy 0.9-mile round-trip trail is accessible to wheelchairs and strollers and is located in the heart of the park, at the base of the highest rock formations.

DESCRIPTION

Leave the parking area, pass the restrooms on the left, and travel south along the Central Garden Trail. Several side trails lead directly to the unusual rock formations, and others lead away from the main trail, but the route is never too far. It is hard to get lost in this park.

Pass the Kissing Camels on the left, defined by a large wall of red rock topped by two formations making the shape of a heart and appearing to kiss. The next rock is to the right, usually blazing in the sun with its white walls: White Rock. To the left is North Gateway Rock. Pass a circular meeting point on the left and save its information kiosks and ample resting spots for the return.

KEY AT-A-GLANCE INFORMATION

LENGTH: 0.9 miles
CONFIGURATION: Loop
DIFFICULTY: Easy
SCENERY: Giant red-rock formations, some grasses, short shrubs
EXPOSURE: Full exposure; some shade in rock formations
TRAFFIC: Heavy
TRAIL SURFACE: Paved
HIKING TIME: 50 minutes
SEASON: All year
ACCESS: Free; open sunrise to sunset
MAPS: USGS Cascade
FACILITIES: Restrooms, picnic facilities; visitor center nearby with interpretive nature displays, classes, tours, and activities; trail is lined with benches and resting spots and loaded with information kiosks that could easily extend a visit here
SPECIAL COMMENTS: Dogs must be leashed. Bikers and equestrians are only permitted on designated trails. Rangers urge visitors not to climb rocks. Climbing is prohibited because, throughout the years, several fatal accidents have occurred.

Directions ⟶

From Denver, take I-25 south to Colorado Springs. Take exit 146, turn right onto Garden of the Gods Road, then turn left onto 30th Street into Garden of the Gods Park. Turn right on Gateway Road, right again on Juniper Way Loop, and left into the north main parking lot.

GPS Trailhead Coordinates

UTM Zone (WGS84)   13S
Easting   0510420
Northing   4303340
Latitude   N 38.878855°
Longitude   W 104.879870°

N

| 0 | 0.05 | 0.1 |
mile

Main Parking Lot

Kissing Camels

Gate Rock

North Gateway Rock

White Rock

Signature Rock

Juniper Way

Juniper Way

Sentinel Rock (Twin Spires)

Pulpit Rock

South Gateway Rock

Cathedral Rock

Gateway Rd.

Three Graces Rock

To visitor center and Colorado Springs

Garden Dr.

Juniper Way

8,500
8,000
7,500
7,000
6,500
6,000
5,500
5,000
4,500

FEET

0.2   0.4   0.6   0.8   0.9

MILES

Study the many large, interesting rock formations, such as this heavenly looking variety, along Perkins Central Garden Trail.

The paved concrete of Central Garden Trail is a subtle mix of reds. At the first fork in the trail, bear right. Pass Signature Rock, then Sentinel Rock (also known as Twin Spires) and move through the unique blend of juniper trees, small spruce trees, brush, and prairie grasses. Loop around, travel beside the road for a short time, and pass Pulpit Rock to the left. Keep right to pass Three Graces and then Cathedral Rock. On the immediate right is South Gateway Rock. Turn right after traveling the length of the western side of South Gateway Rock and head back to the trailhead.

NEARBY ATTRACTIONS

Other Colorado Springs area hikes, including nearby Red Rock Canyon Open Space: **springsgov.com/parks**.

54 NORTH CHEYENNE CAÑON PARK: LOWER COLUMBINE TRAIL

KEY AT-A-GLANCE INFORMATION

LENGTH: 2 miles
CONFIGURATION: Out-and-back
DIFFICULTY: Easy
SCENERY: Canyon, scrub oak, red-rock formations, pine trees
EXPOSURE: Shaded
TRAFFIC: Moderate
TRAIL SURFACE: Dirt
HIKING TIME: 50 minutes
SEASON: All year
ACCESS: Free. Park hours: May 1–October 31, 5 a.m.–11 p.m.; November 1–April 30, 5 a.m.–9 p.m.
MAPS: USGS Colorado Springs, Manitou Springs
FACILITIES: Restrooms, picnic facilities, Starsmore Discovery Center with nature displays, classes, tours, and activities
SPECIAL COMMENTS: Dogs must be leashed. Bikers and equestrians are allowed.

IN BRIEF

The Lower Columbine Trail makes its way up the canyon from behind the Starsmore Discovery Center to Middle Columbine Trail (near the road) to Upper Columbine Trail (near Helen Hunt Falls). The Lower Columbine Trail, featured here, leaves behind the tranquil Starsmore Discovery Center and makes its way 1 mile up the road from the main park gate.

DESCRIPTION

Leave behind the Starsmore Discovery Center. You can either go through the building or take either trail around the perimeter. The trail follows North Cheyenne Cañon Road well into the park. On the left, pass covered picnic tables and restrooms. The trail eventually meets up with a dirt road; continue straight.

Views of Cheyenne Cañon State Park are dominated by massive red-rock formations similar to those seen at Garden of the Gods.

Continue and pass a water-storage unit to the right. Also on the right—within hearing distance—is a small creek with a waterfall. Social trails lead down to the creek, but stay on the wide, well-maintained main trail, which is heavily wooded with tall scrub oaks and pine trees. Pass a series of man-made waterfalls and continue a steady ascent.

GPS Trailhead Coordinates

UTM Zone (WGS84) 13S
Easting   0511723
Northing 4293378
Latitude N 38.789065°
Longitude W 104.865018°

Directions

From Denver, take I-25 south to Colorado Springs. Exit onto CO 24 going west, then turn left onto 21st Street, which turns into Cresta Road. Turn right on Cheyenne Boulevard, drive to the entrance of Cheyenne Cañon Park, and park at the Starsmore Discovery Center.

This hike begins right behind the Starsmore Discovery Center. Be sure to visit its interpretive displays or visit with a volunteer.

In the afternoon, the trail becomes shaded because the canyon walls hide the sun. Pass another picnic area on the right. To the left is a small cave where fires have obviously been stoked because ash burns are all along the rock ceiling. At the sign that points the trail to the left, be sure to go left. A wider trail goes right, but it is a gated entrance to a picnic area. The trail steadily ascends. In steeper areas, stairs are placed into the hillside and some small switchbacks.

You'll travel along the main road for most of this hike, but it never really feels like you are on the road. The trail crests and follows along an area where the hillside is very steep with drop-offs on the right. A missed step here can be dangerous. After the crest, the trail begins to descend before it climbs once more. You'll be able to see the road now. You're still pretty secluded, though, and the hillside is heavily forested. Cross the concrete bridge over the stream and then cross the road to the Middle Columbine Trail, or turn around and head back.

NEARBY ATTRACTIONS

Try the other North Cheyenne Cañon Park trails and other Colorado Springs area hikes, including nearby Stratton Open Space: **springsgov.com/parks.**

PIKE NATIONAL FOREST: DEVIL'S HEAD FIRE LOOKOUT 55

IN BRIEF

The steep staircase that leads to the Devil's Head fire lookout tower is the highlight of the hike. The 143 steps get the best hikers huffing and puffing. The reward at the top is a unique glimpse at a working lookout, one of only 18 that remain in Colorado, the only one staffed by a paid employee. (The remaining 17 are not all in use, and one is available for rent.) Forest Service rangers have scanned for fires in Pike National Forest looking through binoculars for smoke since 1912. It isn't unheard of for veteran rangers to spot more than ten fires in one season.

DESCRIPTION

When you leave the parking lot, pass the benches and concrete patio, and climb the concrete stairs that mark the beginning of the hike. Pine and aspen trees and plenty of places to sit and relax line the trail. Nearby Rampart Range Recreation Area and the 100 miles of off-road motorcycle trails supply the occasional buzz of motorcycles.

Dense trees along the trail create an enchanting effect. Pass a bench. Begin a switchback that includes a small, sturdy footbridge about ten feet long. Continue up another switchback and pass two large benches.

KEY AT-A-GLANCE INFORMATION

LENGTH: 3 miles

CONFIGURATION: Out-and-back

DIFFICULTY: Moderate

SCENERY: Evergreen and aspen forest; fire lookout tower, views

EXPOSURE: Mostly shaded

TRAFFIC: Heavy

TRAIL SURFACE: Dirt; tree roots, loose rocks; large staircase

HIKING TIME: 1.5 hours

SEASON: April–November

ACCESS: Free; open sunrise to sunset

MAPS: USGS Devil's Head

FACILITIES: Picnic tables, water spigot, outhouse

SPECIAL COMMENTS: Dogs must be leashed. Foot traffic only; no bikes; horses allowed but discouraged. Do not climb stairs to the tower during lightning. Forestry officials limit the number of people in the tower at one time. On most days from April–November, the tower is staffed 9:30 a.m.–6 p.m. A campground is at the trailhead, and the ranger says that bears are sighted every night.

Directions

From Denver, take C 470 to US 85 and travel south to Sedalia. In Sedalia, turn right off of US 85 onto CO 67 and head west 10 miles on CO 67 to Rampart Range Road. Go left, traveling south 9.25 miles on this well-maintained dirt road to the trailhead parking.

GPS Trailhead Coordinates

UTM Zone (WGS84)   13S

Easting   0491000

Northing   4346530

Latitude   N 39.268066°

Longitude   W 105.104331°

N

0   0.05   0.1
mile

To
Sedalia

Rampart Range Rd.

P

PIKE
NATIONAL FOREST

To
Deckers

To
Zinn
Overlook

Devil's Head
Lookout

Devil's
Head

FEET

10,000
9,500
9,000
8,500
8,000
7,500
7,000
6,500
6,000

0.25   0.5   0.75   1   1.25   1.5

MILES

A unique sight indeed—the Devil's Head fire lookout.

At the halfway mark, just beyond the large rock, look toward the plains for expansive views of the open prairie. Pass another set of benches; take in the view. Switchback again and pass another set of large rock outcrops.

Look out for the "road apples" in the trail left by mules used to pack supplies to the Forest Service ranger. Pass more benches and a forest-fire information sign.

At 1.2 miles, bear right at a fork in the road and head toward Devil's Head lookout tower. The left turn is an optional, adventurous 0.75-mile side trip to the Zinn Overlook. Continue past the ranger's cabin, more benches, an outhouse, and information signs. The ranger and his wife live in the cabin at the base of the tower. They get groceries once a week and have no running water or sewer.

A steep staircase takes you the final 143 steps to the tower. The lookout tower, which is named on the National Register of Historic Places, perches at 9,748 feet. The massive granite rock outcrop that Devil's Head is named for cannot be seen from the tower because the tower actually sits on top of the outcrop, at the highest point of Devil's Head Mountain. The best views of Devil's Head are actually from Woodland Park.

Once at the tower, chat with the ranger about his curious statistics, such as the youngest (2) to the oldest (90) visitors to reach the tower. On a clear day, the visibility extends more than 100 miles in every direction. The panorama includes Denver, Castle Rock, Sedalia, and 11 of Colorado's fourteeners. From here, turn around and head down the stairs, back to the trailhead.

NEARBY ATTRACTIONS

Pike National Forest Trails and Dutch Fred Trail, Jackson Creek Road, Flat Rocks Overlook: fs.fed.us/r2/psicc/recreation/trails.

56 PIKE NATIONAL FOREST: WIGWAM TRAIL

KEY AT-A-GLANCE INFORMATION

LENGTH: 9.34 miles

CONFIGURATION: Out-and-back

DIFFICULTY: Moderate

SCENERY: Dense evergreen and aspen forest; wetlands

EXPOSURE: Shaded

TRAFFIC: Light

TRAIL SURFACE: Dirt; tree roots, loose rocks

HIKING TIME: 4.5 hours

SEASON: May–October (open all year)

ACCESS: Free; open sunrise to sunset

MAPS: USGS Green Mountain, Cheesman Lake, Windy Peak

FACILITIES: None

SPECIAL COMMENTS: Wilderness regulations apply to this hike in the Lost Creek Wilderness Area. Dogs must be leashed; campers must have permits; horses are permitted but restricted; no motorized or wheeled vehicles, so no bikes. Weather conditions tend to be colder and wetter in the higher elevations of this hike.

IN BRIEF

The drive to the trailhead takes hikers through massive square miles of burned forest that were torched in Colorado's largest wildfire, the Haymen Fire (2002). In contrast, the Wigwam Trail testifies to what did survive. Lush, green, heavy vegetation and tall evergreen trees are quite a relief. Off of the beaten path, the trail is lightly used, and hikers do not encounter many other humans.

DESCRIPTION

The official trailhead (Wigwam Trail #609) can be found at the end of the lower parking lot where the road turns around. Sign in at the trailhead log sheet. Hike across Wigwam Creek and then cross it again. Here, you officially enter the Lost Creek Wilderness Area. Cross primitive rock bridges as you follow the Wigwam Creek drainage uphill.

The trail heads northwest along Wigwam Creek and rises with a moderate ascending grade. Evergreen trees and low growth mark the landscape for several miles, following the creek's drainage, before the trail opens up. Travel into lush meadows as the creek flows

GPS Trailhead Coordinates

UTM Zone (WGS84) 13S

Easting   0469510

Northing   4343920

Latitude   N 39.244058°

Longitude W 105.353329°

Directions

From Denver, take I-70 west to C 470 to US 285, traveling west for 23 miles to Pine Junction. Turn left at the town of Pine Junction onto CO 126, toward Pine and Buffalo Creek. Drive 21.8 miles on CO 126. Turn left, traveling south on FS 211, which leads toward Cheesman Reservoir. Travel 2 miles and bear right at the sign pointing to Goose Creek. Drive 1.1 miles until you reach a fork, bear right on FS 560, and bear right at the next fork staying on FS 560. Drive 4 miles to the trailhead signs, turn left at the signs, and drive 1.3 miles to the trailhead.

Lush landscape is found frequently along the Wigwam Trail.

into numerous beaver ponds. Some of these beaver ponds are rather large. Small aspen trees along the trail have been gnawed down by beavers and used to dam up Wigwam Creek.

This area is called Wigwam Park. The last stretch to the park has several short, steep, rocky sections. Continue straight at the intersection with Goose Creek Trail, and just to the west of there, pass the intersection with Rolling Creek Trail. Continue, cross the creek again, and enter a grove of tall aspens.

The hike ascends, crosses the creek one last time, and ends in a high saddle at the end of the mountain valley, after the meadows and before the descent into East Lost Park. Turn around here and retrace your steps back to the trailhead. You can continue on from the turnaround point, since Wigwam Trail has approximately 6 more miles of trail.

NEARBY ATTRACTIONS

Pike National Forest Trails, Goose Creek Trail (# 619), Rolling Creek Trail (# 663), and Brookside-McCurdy Trail: **fs.fed.us/r2/psicc/recreation/trails.**

PINE VALLEY RANCH PARK: PINE VALLEY RANCH LOOP   57

IN BRIEF

Visitors to Pine Valley Ranch Park can hike the trails, fish from the pond piers, ice-skate in the winter, enjoy observatory programs, and connect to Pike National Forest for additional recreation. Pine Valley Ranch Park enjoys a unique blend of historic and natural features, such as the fact that Narrow Gauge Trail, part of the loop, follows the original railroad bed.

DESCRIPTION

At the trailhead is the Pine Valley Ranch Depot. Stop here to read the information signs and pick up a park map. Start hiking west on Narrow Gauge Trail. The wide trail leads you through dense willows along the North Fork of the South Platte River. Turn left onto Buck Gulch Trail and cross over the river via a wooden bridge.

Continue south on Buck Gulch Trail; pass the North Fork View Trail turnoff. A set of restrooms and a covered picnic area are here. You can now see Pine Lake on the left. Follow the trail as it narrows and begins to climb into the hills away from the lake. Turn left onto Strawberry Jack Trail and travel into Pike National Forest, continuing the steady ascent.

KEY AT-A-GLANCE INFORMATION

LENGTH: 3.2 miles
CONFIGURATION: Loop
DIFFICULTY: Moderate
SCENERY: Scenic vistas, forest, lake, river
EXPOSURE: Mostly shaded
TRAFFIC: Moderate
TRAIL SURFACE: Dirt, loose rocks
HIKING TIME: 1.5 hours
SEASON: All year
ACCESS: Free; open 1 hour before sunrise to 1 hour after sunset
MAPS: USGS Pine
FACILITIES: Restrooms, group picnic shelters, Pine Valley Ranch Depot information kiosk, observatory
SPECIAL COMMENTS: Dogs must be leashed. Portions of the trail are hiker only. The park has some handicap-accessible facilities and hiking areas. Observatory programs are scheduled through the Lookout Mountain Nature Center at (303) 526-0594. Reserve a shelter for an event at (303) 271-5925.

Directions

From Denver, take I-70 west to C 470 south to US 285 south to Pine Junction. Turn left off of US 285, going southeast onto Pine Valley Road (CR 126), and continue 5.8 miles to the town of Pine. Turn right onto Crystal Lake Road and follow it 1.22 miles to the trailhead.

GPS Trailhead Coordinates

UTM Zone (WGS84)   13S
Easting   0470127
Northing   4361946
Latitude   N 39.406506°
Longitude   W 105.346980°

N

| 0 | 0.1 | 0.2 |

mile

Crystal Lake Rd.

Baehr
Lodge

N. Fork S. Platte River

Pine Valley
Ranch Depot

Pine Lake Loop

North Fork View Trl.

Pine Lake

Crystal Lake Rd.

P

To Pike →

Pine Lake Loop

Narrow Gauge Trl.

Buck Gulch Trl.

Park View Trl.

PINE VALLEY
RANCH PARK

Buck Gulch

Buck Gulch Trl.

Strawberry Jack Trl.

PIKE
NATIONAL
FOREST

FEET							
8,500							
8,000				→			
7,500							
7,000							
6,500							
6,000							
5,500							
5,000							
4,500							

| | 0.5 | 1 | 1.5 | 2 | 2.5 | 3 | 3.2 |

MILES

Cute but wild chipmunks, such as this native, frequent the area around Pine Valley Ranch Park.

The trail shows evidence of the destruction of forest fires. Burned trees and telltale signs of new growth signify the rebirth of a forest. At 1.25 miles, you reach Park View Trail. Turn left and reach the highest point of this hike, just beyond the intersection. Begin to descend and pass a bench halfway down the hill. This is a good place to take in the view: Pine Lake, the observatory, and Baehr Lodge, with a large rock outcrop as a backdrop. The lodge was built in 1927 and is now listed on the National Register of Historic Places.

Well-constructed stairs make the steep descent a little easier as the trail winds toward the lake. Turn left onto Pine Lake Loop. Keep your eyes open for wildlife that may include beavers, especially as you approach the wetlands at the west edge of the lake. Complete the Pine Lake Loop, going clockwise, and cross back over the river to the trailhead.

NEARBY ATTRACTIONS

Other Jefferson County area hikes and Pine Valley Ranch Park connector trails: **jeffco.us/openspace.**

58 REYNOLDS OPEN SPACE PARK: RAVEN'S ROOST OXEN DRAW LOOP

KEY AT-A-GLANCE INFORMATION

LENGTH: 3.7 miles

CONFIGURATION: Loop

DIFFICULTY: Moderate

SCENERY: Wide variety of evergreens: ponderosa, blue spruce, Douglas fir, alpine fir

EXPOSURE: Mostly shaded

TRAFFIC: Moderate

TRAIL SURFACE: Dirt, rocky in sections

HIKING TIME: 1.75 hours

SEASON: All year

ACCESS: Free; open 1 hour before sunrise to 1 hour after sunset

MAPS: USGS Platte Canyon, Pine

FACILITIES: Outhouse, picnic tables

SPECIAL COMMENTS: Dogs must be leashed. No bikes.

IN BRIEF

Raven's Roost Oxen Draw Loop is a straightforward up-and-down hike with an additional steep climb to the Eagle View Trail Overlook. Enjoy a great view of the South Platte area from this vantage point. An interpretive trail identifies plants along this diverse trail.

DESCRIPTION

From the parking area, begin to hike on the Raven's Roost Trail and turn right when the outhouse comes into sight. Raven's Roost Trail and Elkhorn Interpretive Trail merge for a short time. Pick up an interpretive trail guide at a post along the trail. Follow Elkhorn Interpretive Trail and climb several switchbacks until Raven's Roost Trail breaks off to the right. Raven's Roost turns into a Forest Service road for a while as the route follows the steep roadbed along the ridgeline.

Follow Raven's Roost Trail as it separates from the Forest Service road and begins to descend, dropping down to a small creek crossing. At the next trail intersection, turn right onto Eagle's View Trail. This trail is steep and leads hikers to a ridgeline and small meadow with a marvelous vantage point. To the south are views of Pikes Peak and Rampart Range. Turn around and head back on Eagle's

GPS Trailhead Coordinates

UTM Zone (WGS84) 13S

Easting   0479481

Northing   4368386

Latitude   N 39.464808°

Longitude   W 105.238531°

Directions

From Denver, take I-70 west to C 470 south to US 285 south to Conifer. Travel through Conifer to Foxton Road. Go left on Foxton Road for 5.3 miles to Reynolds Open Space and a large, dirt parking lot on the south side of the road.

58 Reynolds Open Space Park:
Raven's Roost Oxen Draw Loop

N

0   0.1   0.2
mile

To
Conifer

Foxton Rd.

Kennedy Gulch

Foxton Rd.

REYNOLDS
OPEN SPACE
PARK

Raven's Roost Trl.

Raven's Roost
Trl.

Hummingbird
Trl.

Elkhorn Interpretive Trl.

Forest Service Rd.

Songbird Trl.

Oxen Draw Trl.

Eagle's View Trl.

Eagle's
View

9,000

8,500

8,000

7,500

7,000

6,500

6,000

5,500

5,000

FEET

1   2   3   3.7

MILES

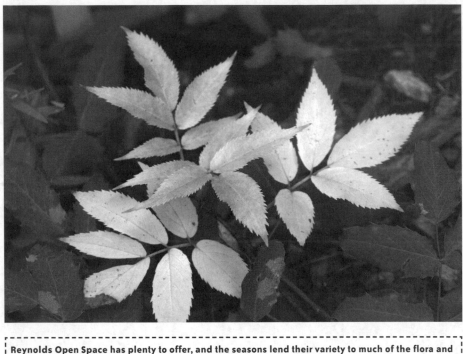

Reynolds Open Space has plenty to offer, and the seasons lend their variety to much of the flora and fauna along the trail.

View Trail, to the intersection of Eagle's View, Raven's Roost, and Oxen Draw Trails. Turn right onto Oxen Draw Trail and cross the stream a number of times. This trail follows the ravine through dense forest and brings hikers back to Elkhorn Interpretive Trail. Turn right onto Elkhorn Interpretive Trail and continue past the next intersection. Come to a bench placed at the edge of a relaxing meadow filled with wildflowers in the summer. Turn left onto Songbird Trail and head back to the trailhead.

NEARBY ATTRACTIONS

Other Jefferson County area hikes, including Songbird Trail and Hummingbird Trail in Reynolds Open Space. Visit the Web site at **jeffco.us/openspace**.

ROXBOROUGH STATE PARK: SOUTH RIM TRAIL   59

IN BRIEF

Roxborough State Park is a Colorado Natural Area and a National Natural Landmark. The park offers two main hiking areas: Fountain Valley and South Rim. Fountain Valley Trail has a dramatic trailhead and a big parking lot. South Rim Trail has the same scenery and fewer people. The remarkable geology of this area is largely represented by the Fountain Formation. These red rocks jettison from the earth, erupting from the green valley.

DESCRIPTION

From the parking area, drop down below the road, go 100 yards, and cross a bridge, starting out on Willow Creek Trail going southeast. Take a left at the intersection with Willow Creek Trail, onto South Rim Trail, and start ascending. To the right you'll see some of the red-rock formations, primarily the Fountain Formation, that dominate this area. As the trail climbs and the views expand, you will have constant views of these amazing rows of tilted rocks.

When the trail begins to switchback, hikers may begin to notice the scrub oaks, yucca plants, sagebrush, and cacti. The trail continues

KEY AT-A-GLANCE INFORMATION

LENGTH: 2.3 miles
CONFIGURATION: Balloon
DIFFICULTY: Moderate
SCENERY: Jutting rock formations, foothill views
EXPOSURE: No shade
TRAFFIC: Moderate
TRAIL SURFACE: Hard-packed dirt
HIKING TIME: 1.5 hours
SEASON: All year
ACCESS: $6 or state parks pass; open sunrise to sunset
MAPS: USGS Kassler
FACILITIES: Visitor center, restrooms, pay phone
SPECIAL COMMENTS: No dogs, no horses, and no bikes. Park hours change with the seasons and are posted in the park and at parks.state.co.us. Bears, mountain lions, and rattlesnakes are common in this park.

Directions

From Denver, take C 470 south to the Wadsworth Boulevard (CO 121) exit. Take Wadsworth Boulevard left, going south for 4.3 miles, then turn left on Waterton Road. After 1.7 miles, turn right on Rampart Range Road and travel 4 miles, then take a left on Roxborough Park Road. Follow the signs to the park. Pay your fee and cross through the official park gate and entrance. The South Rim parking lot has only about 10 spaces and is the first parking area on your left.

GPS Trailhead Coordinates

UTM Zone (WGS84)   13S
Easting   0494577
Northing   4364232
Latitude   N 39.427605°
Longitude   W 105.063008°

ROXBOROUGH
STATE PARK

Visitor
Center

Roxborough Park Rd.

Willow Creek

To
Denver

N. Brightwater Trl.

Willow Creek Trl.

Willow Creek Trl.

South Rim Trl.

South Rim
Overlook

Carpenter Peak
Trl.

Roxborough Dr.

Willow Creek

South Rim Trl.

N   0   0.1   0.2
mile

FEET

8,500
8,000
7,500
7,000
6,500
6,000
5,500
5,000
4,500

0.5   1   1.5   2   2.3

MILES

its gentle ascent, continually curving to the right.

Once you reach the ridgetop, the South Rim Overlook, the trail starts curving to the left instead. New red-rock formations dot the view. A light-yellow ridge east of the Fountain Formation is the Lyons Formation. The Dakota Hogback Ridge, another rock formation, can be seen in the distance with the same red rocks in a jettison row.

At the next intersection, with a social trail leading to a scenic overlook, keep going straight on South Rim Trail. Begin to descend as the trail starts to switchback, then deposits you into the rock formations. Continue straight at the intersection with Carpenter Peak Trail, staying on South Rim Trail. Look out for the intersection with Willow Creek Trail, which comes up fast and forks in from behind. You'll take a right here; a left turn will take you to the visitor center on the southwest portion of Willow Creek Trail. It's easy to miss if you are absorbed in the rock formations. At the next intersection with South Rim Trail, take a left to complete the balloon and return to the trailhead.

NEARBY ATTRACTIONS

Within Roxborough State Park are five additional hiking trails: Fountain Valley Overlook, Lyons Overlook, Willow Creek, Fountain Valley, and Carpenter Peak. Waterton Canyon and Sharptail Ridge Open Space are also close. Visit **parks. state.co.us/parks/roxborough** for more information.

60 WATERTON CANYON RECREATION AREA: WATERTON CANYON

KEY AT-A-GLANCE INFORMATION

LENGTH: 8 miles

CONFIGURATION: Out-and-back

DIFFICULTY: Moderate

SCENERY: Foothills, South Platte River, grassy areas, river habitat, cliff walls

EXPOSURE: Shaded by canyon walls and cottonwoods along the river

TRAFFIC: Heavy

TRAIL SURFACE: Smooth and hard-packed dirt

HIKING TIME: 4 hours

SEASON: All year

ACCESS: Free; open sunrise to sunset

MAPS: USGS Kassler and Platte Canyon

FACILITIES: Restrooms (handicap accessible), picnic facilities, bike rack, pay phone

SPECIAL COMMENTS: To protect wildlife, no dogs are allowed. The parking lot accommodates 150 cars and 20 horse trailers, so crowded conditions may exist, especially on the early portion of the trail.

IN BRIEF

Waterton Canyon serves as a trailhead for the 475-mile-long Colorado Trail. This is a long walk south to the Durango area, yet Waterton Canyon allows hikers to walk as far as they please and turn around. The featured hike travels 4 miles into the canyon as it follows the South Platte River into the mountains. This user-friendly hike is an enjoyable outing.

DESCRIPTION

Cross Waterton Road and find the sign COL-ORADO TRAIL TRAILHEAD. The information board and trail marker are on a short dirt trail a few hundred feet beyond Waterton Road. Head west as the trail quickly turns into an asphalt road that carries you along the west side of the old Kassler water treatment facility. Almost immediately, the asphalt gives way to hard-packed dirt as the road continues beyond the treatment plant and toward the South Platte River. The trail passes through short bushes and tall grasses that line the river. Both covered and uncovered picnic tables as well as outhouses are plentiful along this portion of the trail, so finding a resting spot is never a challenge. The trail also serves as a road for

------

GPS Trailhead Coordinates

UTM Zone (WGS84)   13S

Easting   0491876

Northing   4370999

Latitude   N 39.488559°

Longitude   W 105.094473°

Directions

From Denver, take C 470 south to the Wadsworth Boulevard (CO 121) exit. Take a left, going south on Wadsworth Boulevard, which quickly becomes South Platte Canyon Road. Continue south to West Waterton Road and turn left (east, the only way you can turn onto Waterton). The parking lot is immediately on the left (north) side of West Waterton Road. The trail marker and information post is several hundred feet south of the road.

N

0   0.3   0.6
mile

South Platte Reservoir

South Platte River

W. Waterton Rd.

P

To Denver

Old Kassler water treatment facility

Colorado Trl.

canal

C A N Y O N

W A T E R T O N

Cottonwood Gulch

South Platte River

Goat Mtn.

Horse, shop, and emergency phone

Marston Diversion Dam

Colorado Trl.

8,500

8,000

7,500

7,000

6,500

6,000

5,500

5,000

4,500

FEET

1   2   3   4
MILES

Wildlife is plentiful in Waterton Canyon, as a crane gracefully demonstrates in a marshy wetland.

the water department, although public vehicular access is restricted.

Continue on the trail, which is now a wide, two-lane dirt road with smooth and hard-packed surfaces, shaded by cottonwoods. Plenty of foot, bicycle, and horse traffic exist at this deservedly popular trail. Well maintained with a smooth, continuous slope, the trail closely follows the South Platte River as it winds its way into Waterton Canyon.

Each turn provides new interest to hikers as the trail continues. Beaver dams dot the waterways along the trail; some hikers may be lucky enough to see beavers swimming, especially later in the day. One of the many bends in the trail brings hikers underneath two large water-supply pipes to a small dam. Following the aqueduct are impressive cliffs that rise on the north side of the trail. At this point, the trail is in prime Rocky Mountain bighorn sheep territory. While scanning the rocks for bighorn sheep, don't forget to watch the riverbanks as well. Blue herons nest here and can be seen fishing for their next meal. Anglers regularly fly-fish in this part of the river.

The trail crosses through terrain that is less rocky and passes an unmarked trail that branches off to the northwest. Waterton Canyon tends to lure you from bend to bend, so it is important to be attentive to the time and weather. The canyon walls limit the amount of sky that can be seen, so storm clouds tend to surprise hikers. The walls also block the sun as it begins to set.

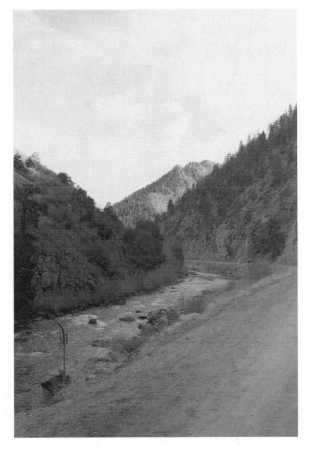

The South Platte River and the gentle hills of Waterton Canyon.

Continue along to another water diversion structure. At this point, there is an emergency telephone, house, and mechanical shop used by water maintenance personnel. Eventually hikers arrive at Marston Diversion Dam, where the sheet of water flowing over the dam highlights the hike. Turn around here to hike 4 miles back to your car.

Some hikers may want to continue up the canyon to where the trail intersects the beginning of the Colorado Trail. The Colorado Trail stretches all the way to Durango for those prepared and ambitious overnight hikers who want to trek several hundred miles.

NEARBY ATTRACTIONS

Colorado Trail: **coloradotrail.org.**

APPENDIXES
AND INDEX

APPENDIX A:
OUTDOOR STORES

Army and Navy Surplus Store—Denver
armysurplusforless.com
(888) 804-LESS (5377)
7560 Pecos Street
Denver, CO 80221
(303) 426-0488

Englewood
3524 South Broadway
Englewood, CO 80113
(303) 789-1827

Arvada Army Navy Surplus
arvadasurplus.com
5701 Olde Wadsworth Blvd.
Arvada, CO 80002
(303) 424-5434

Backpacker's Pantry
backpackerspantry.com
6350 Gunpark Drive
Boulder, CO 80303
(303) 581-0581; (800) 641-0500

Bike-N-Hike
1136 Main Street
Longmont, CO 80501
(303) 772-5105

Boulder Army Store
boulderarmystore.com
1545 Pearl Street
Boulder, CO 80303
(303) 442-7616

Hiking Hut
110 East Elkhorn Avenue
Estes Park, CO 80517
(970) 586-0708

JAX Outdoor Gear
jaxmercantile.com
1200 North College Avenue
Fort Collins, CO 80524
(970) 221-0544; (800) 336-8314

**Little Mountain Outfitters,
Outdoor Gear for Kids**
littlemountainoutfitters.com
1136 Spruce Street
Boulder, CO 80302
(303) 443-1757

McGuckin Hardware
mcguckin.com
2525 Arapahoe Avenue
Boulder, CO 80303
(303) 443-1822

Mountain Sports
2835 Pearl Street
Boulder, CO 80302
(303) 442-8355

Neptune Mountaineering
neptunemountaineering.com
633 South Broadway, Suite A
Boulder, CO 80305
(303) 499-8866; (888) 499-8866

The North Face
thenorthface.com
1711 29th Street
Boulder, CO 80301
(303) 499-1731

Outdoor Divas
outdoordivas.com
(866) 449-DIVA (3482)
1133 Pearl Street
Boulder, CO 80302
(303) 449-DIVA (3482)

Denver
2717 East Third Avenue
Denver, CO 80206
(303) 320-DIVA (3482)

Patagonia
patagonia.com
1431 15th Street
Denver, CO 80202
(303) 446-9500

Boulder
1212 Pearl Street
Boulder, CO 80302
(720) 479-2387

REI
rei.com
1416 Platte Street
Denver, CO 80202
(303) 756-3100

Lakewood
5375 South Wadsworth Boulevard
Lakewood, CO 80123
(303) 932-0600

Englewood
9637 East County Line Road
Englewood, CO 80112
(303) 858-1726

Boulder
1789 28th Street
Boulder, CO 80301
(303) 583-9970

Fort Collins
4025 South College Avenue
Fort Collins, CO 80525
(970) 223-0123

Colorado Springs
1376 East Woodmen Road
Colorado Springs, CO 80920
(719) 260-1455

Trailridge Outfitters
358 East Elkhorn Avenue
Estes Park, CO 80517
(970) 586-4595

Large Sporting Goods Chain Stores:

Christy Sports
christysports.com

Sports Authority
sportsauthority.com

APPENDIX B:
MAP SHOPS

Boulder Army Store
boulderarmystore.com
1545 Pearl Street
Boulder, CO 80303
(303) 442-7616

Boulder Map Gallery
bouldermapgallery.com
1718 13th Street
Boulder, CO 80302
(303) 444-1406

BikeDenver
bikedenver.org/maps

DeLorme
delorme.com

Golden Outfitters
17211 West 16th Place
Golden, CO 80401
(303) 279-4140

Google Maps
maps.google.com

Indian Peaks Ace Hardware
74 Highway 119 South
Nederland, CO 80466
(303) 258-3132

JAX Outdoor Gear
jaxmercantile.com
1200 North College Avenue
Fort Collins, CO 80524
(970) 221-0544

MacVan Map Co.
macvanmaps.com
929 West Colorado Avenue
Colorado Springs, CO 80905
(719) 636-9300; (800) 473-6277

MapQuest
mapquest.com

Maptech,Inc.
maptech.com

McGuckin Hardware
mcguckin.com
2525 Arapahoe Avenue
Boulder, CO 80303
(303) 443-1822

Microsoft Mapblast
mapblast.com

National Geographic MapMachine
nationalgeographic.com/
mapmachine

National Geographic Maps
nationalgeographic.com/maps

APPENDIX B:
MAP SHOPS (CONTINUED)

The North Face
thenorthface.com
1711 29th Street
Boulder, CO 80301
(303) 499-1731

Offroute
offroute.com

REI
rei.com
All local REI stores

Tattered Cover
tatteredcover.com
2526 East Colfax Avenue
Denver, CO 80206
(303) 322-7727

LoDo
1628 16th Street
Denver, CO 80202
(303) 436-1070

Highlands Ranch
9315 Dorchester Street
Highlands Ranch, CO 80129
(303) 470-7050

Timely Topos
557 Burbank Street
Broomfield, CO 80020
(303) 469-5022

Topo USA
topozone.com

USDA Forest Service
fs.fed.us

Maps by Phone:
(303) 275-5350
(303) 275-5367 (hearing impaired)

*Maps available at all local
agency offices*
United State Geologic Survey
usgs.gov

USGS Map Store
store.usgs.gov

GPS Manufacturers:

Brunton
brunton.com

Garmin
garmin.com

Magellan
magellangps.com

Suunto
suunto.com

APPENDIX C:
AREA HIKING CLUBS

Access Fund
accessfund.org

Active.com
active.com

American Hiking Society
americanhiking.org

American Trails
americantrails.org

America Walks
americawalks.org

Climb the Rockies
climbtherockies.com

Colorado Fourteeners Initiative
coloradofourteeners.org

Colorado Mountain Club
cmc.org

Colorado Trail Foundation
coloradotrail.org

Continental Divide Trail Alliance
cdtrail.org

Fourteeners.org
fourteeners.org

Geocache Resources
geocaching.com

Happy Hikers Club
happyhikersclub.org

Hiking and Backpacking
hikingandbackpacking.com/
coloradoclubs.html

Hiking in Colorado
hikingincolorado.org

Letterboxing
letterboxing.org

Mountain Peaks
mountainpeaks.net

Road Runner Club of America
rrca.org

Rocky Mountain Nature Association
rmna.org

Running Network
runningnetwork.com

Run Walk Jog
runwalkjog.com

Sierra Club
rmc.sierraclub.org
Rocky Mountain Chapter
1536 Wynkoop Street, 4C
Denver, CO 80202
(303) 861-8819

Trails.com
trails.com

Volunteers for Outdoor Colorado
voc.org

INDEX

DEAR CUSTOMERS AND FRIENDS,

SUPPORTING YOUR INTEREST IN OUTDOOR ADVENTURE, travel, and an active lifestyle is central to our operations, from the authors we choose to the locations we detail to the way we design our books. Menasha Ridge Press was incorporated in 1982 by a group of veteran outdoorsmen and professional outfitters. For many years now, we've specialized in creating books that benefit the outdoors enthusiast.

Almost immediately, Menasha Ridge Press earned a reputation for revolutionizing outdoors- and travel-guidebook publishing. For such activities as canoeing, kayaking, hiking, backpacking, and mountain biking, we established new standards of quality that transformed the whole genre, resulting in outdoor-recreation guides of great sophistication and solid content. Menasha Ridge continues to be outdoor publishing's greatest innovator.

The folks at Menasha Ridge Press are as at home on a white-water river or mountain trail as they are editing a manuscript. The books we build for you are the best they can be, because we're responding to your needs. Plus, we use and depend on them ourselves.

We look forward to seeing you on the river or the trail. If you'd like to contact us directly, join in at www.trekalong.com or visit us at www.menasharidge.com. We thank you for your interest in our books and the natural world around us all.

SAFE TRAVELS,

Bob Sehlinger

BOB SEHLINGER
PUBLISHER